SIRENS

SIRENS

INSIDE THE SHADOW WORLD OF FIRST RESPONDERS

MARTIN MCKENZIE-MURRAY

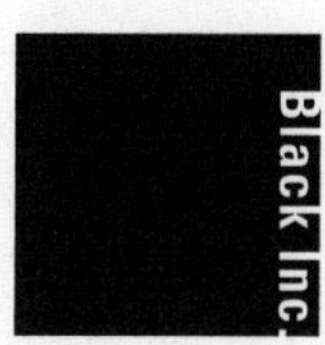

Published by Black Inc.,
an imprint of Schwartz Books Pty Ltd
Wurundjeri Country
22–24 Northumberland Street
Collingwood VIC 3066, Australia
enquiries@blackincbooks.com
www.blackincbooks.com

9781760642877 (paperback)
9781743824597 (ebook)

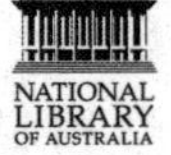

A catalogue record for this book is available from the National Library of Australia

Book design and typesetting by Beau Lowenstern
Cover image: borchee/iStock
Parts of this book first appeared in
The Saturday Paper and *The Monthly*.

Printed in Australia by McPherson's Printing Group.

For those who rush in

If we had a keen vision and feeling of all ordinary human life, it would be like hearing the grass grow and the squirrel's heart beat, and we should die of that roar which lies on the other side of silence.

George Eliot, *Middlemarch*

CONTENTS

Dear reader:

A book about trauma and traumatic work will, necessarily, describe traumatic events. As much as our culture can treat blood, violence and villainy as a form of entertainment, the antidote to this vampiric compulsion, it seems to me, is *not* to throw a blanket over it. Especially in the case of this book: what the subjects have seen has, in different ways, changed who they are.

The book that you now hold also treats in detail the childhoods of these three people – and to a lesser extent my own – and as such stories of domestic and sexual abuse are recounted. So, now you know.

I might add here that something useful may come from reading about these lives: the shock of recognition. In writing this book, but also in fifteen years of journalism, I've frequently found patterns in how individuals respond (or don't) to trauma. One recurring element among the three subjects here, and it's been true of myself also, is the reluctance to seek help. We can too often ignore, rationalise or falsely diminish our pain when help is often not too far away.

SUPPORT SERVICES

Lifeline	lifelinedirect.org.au	13 11 14
Beyond Blue	beyondblue.org.au	1300 22 4636
Phoenix Australia	phoenixaustralia.org	03 9035 5599

Introduction

Ever since I was a young boy, I've experienced variations of the same nightmare. The dreams involve aircraft – planes, usually, but sometimes helicopters. I'm never a passenger, but instead a prophetic witness on the ground, before its destruction.

This awareness, and my recognition of its uselessness, is perhaps the most sinister quality of the dream. My knowledge is impotent, and I submit to the atmosphere of doom and paralysis.

Then comes the demon whine of failing engines. Then the plane stalls and drops from the sky like a dead angel. There is a great roar, the earth shakes, and then comes the fiery rain of debris.

Only once did I bother to record the details of one of these dreams. It was about seven years ago, when my partner was pregnant with our daughter.

On this occasion, uniquely moved to record the dream, I reached over to my bedside table and wrote:

> Day: Saturday. Time: 5.43 am. Stress levels: Okay. Description: British Airways commercial liner. Warped by imagination – plane doesn't have regular engines, but one afterburner. Is taking off. Despite the wicked sound of the engine, appears to be climbing normally. An old friend is watching with me. Orphaned young in waking life. Then the plane slows. Too slow. It stalls, falls. Explosion. Dread. I wake.

My dream-self witnesses mass death and is sometimes mortally threatened by the ensuing inferno. But that's not what lingers. What lingers is the quality of dread – the sticky, black residue that lines my consciousness long after I've woken.

Such dreams have startled me from sleep for nearly forty years now. What element of my unconscious life has remained constant all that time? Or perhaps that was the wrong way to think about it. Could there be some unprocessed memory that was begging for conscious treatment?

—

In 2024, about a month before what I'll call my unravelling, we celebrated my daughter's fifth birthday in a community hall, which we decorated with bright strings of balloons.

I had developed a problem with balloons. I knew by then that the sudden bursting of one was agonising for my nervous system – just as any other sudden noise was and, increasingly, *my own shadow*, which had, in the fulfillment of a terrible cliché, developed the capacity to startle me.

Much of this I kept to myself. But being in a room filled with balloons was an agony of anticipation, and I crept around, hypervigilant, saddened by how distracted I was on this day of celebration.

At the end of my daughter's party came the job of disposing of the balloons, and I was determined to do it myself. The thought of piercing dozens of them didn't thrill me, but assuming control of the job was preferable to allowing someone else to do it.

–

When your child stops breathing, time dilates. Seconds are experienced as long and hysterical days. And there's a wickedly vivid compression of thoughts – thoughts that mark like a tattooist's pen; thoughts that I can't describe here. Enough to say that these are diabolically crowded seconds, in which the bleakest future is both seen and deeply felt.

She choked. On the food I gave her. I was right beside her. I knew she'd put too much in. At first, her expression was one of sweet, innocent confusion. Then alarm. Then her face changed colour. Then there was silence. From her at least. I had her over my knee horizontally, face down, while I called triple zero. How do I unlock my phone? Do I scream for the neighbours' help? I was alone, my partner at work. *How long did we have?*

I slammed her back. Nothing. I slammed again. Nothing. How much force is too much? How much is too little? I thought about the baby first-aid course I took before she was born. I thought about the mannequin and its hard plastic flesh.

The emergency service was on speaker now.

"Don't hit her back," they said. I wondered how I'd managed to make contact with them – did *I* call them? Of course, I was the only one there.

Only months earlier had I called triple zero for the first time. I'd stepped off my tram and found an old lady had fallen, her head split open. Blood was splashed on her bag of grapes. I put pressure on the wound, shielded her from the sun, held her hand. She was in shock; she was repeating herself. A sweet woman. After a while she improved. She wanted to get up; she wanted to go home. I told her an ambulance was on its way, and their advice was for her to stay here. She obliged. I asked about her life, got her address for the paramedics.

But what I was thinking about with my daughter over my knee was how long that ambulance for the old lady had taken to arrive – about forty-five minutes. But I thought: *surely*, they triage? As I held the woman's hand, the operator had asked me a lot of questions – answers to which were surely fed into a system of prioritisation. So maybe *this* ambulance would be faster? Surely, *surely*.

It wasn't needed. I thrust my index finger in her mouth, down her throat and scooped out the food. Was that all of it? It didn't seem like enough. But she was screaming now – a good sign. I went back in, scooped out some more. Our two cats pounced on it, and their opportunism and obliviousness seemed faintly obscene.

I was holding my daughter's hand now. She recovered quickly. I didn't. Paramedics called me again, and falteringly I told them I didn't think they were needed anymore. But I could barely speak. I was shaking, crying, while my daughter was asking for a book. Unlike the cats', her obliviousness was cherished. How much time had passed? I couldn't tell you. After my partner returned from work, I spent much of the afternoon trembling and experiencing sudden bursts of weeping.

For many months, I had intrusive memories, which I worsened by elaborately transforming them into worst-case scenarios. The poisonous thing about intrusive memories is that they introduce not merely an image, but the *feeling* of that moment.

I drank more, and developed an intense interest in space exploration.

—

The supermoon lived at the end of our street, or it did briefly one evening, and in the days before I'd excitedly primed my daughter for its appearance. I scooped her up, ignored her protests and walked out into the middle of our street.

Her reluctance thawed, and she charmingly mistook the streetlights for our supermoon. But then, unmistakably, there it was: bright, plump and enthroned just above the horizon.

"I get step?" she asked. She wanted to climb and touch it.

Perhaps seven or eight months had passed since the incident. The choking. We were still in Melbourne's Covid lockdown, and I found great pleasure in showing my daughter the moon and the stars. As I did in writing to astronauts, and to a man who had designed a sculpture of one that was placed on the moon to commemorate those who had died in the pursuit of space exploration.

The sculpture is still up there now, along with the abandoned moon buggies and ziplocked bags of shit. Along with the flags and golf balls and long faded family photos that astronauts left behind.

—

My own diagnosis of PTSD came years after I began work on this book. After years of hearing about the symptoms of others, it became harder to deny my own. But instead of making this admission and seeking help, I simply recalibrated my denial: instead of denying that I likely had PTSD, I now denied its importance and severity.

I was labouring naively under the belief that the symptoms would improve the more time passed. I was humbled to learn that the opposite was true. Things worsened. The intrusive memories slightly improved, but everything else got worse: the irritability, the hypervigilance, the insomnia. So too the nightmares and the vast volumes of sweat, so much that I could replace my singlet several times a night. So often did I interpret as an imminent heart attack what I now realise to have been severe panic attacks that I took to patrolling the street of the nearest GP, just so I'd be close to medics if I collapsed from cardiac arrest.

By now, I'd developed tics – violent twitches of my face and arms – and exhaustion was constant. When the nervous system is continually aroused in the mistaken belief that you, or a loved one, are dying, the electric suffusion of cortisol eventually retreats and leaves you beached upon a rocky shore. Our primal flight or fight instincts are not meant to be triggered daily, nor our bodies flooded with severe hormones, and there's a commensurate low after the high of their deployment. A nervous system that's either permanently adrenalised or recovering from its arousal doesn't leave much left, and "it's exhausting pretending you're normal", as Peter, the paramedic in this book, told me when I eventually shared my diagnosis with him.

There is nothing ennobling about PTSD. It does not enhance you. The world and its possibilities narrow cruelly to perceived threats. You're more irritable, more sensitive, more caustic and more self-concerned. You can become less generous, less warm, less resilient. You may become dimly aware of a slow frosting of your soul – a transformation into a colder, pricklier and frailer person than you'd like to be.

–

I began a course of Eye Movement Desensitisation and Reprocessing therapy (EMDR) in 2024. Before I did, there was a lot of preparatory work. Most of this involved my therapist enquiring about my past – establishing my "history". One aim of this excavation was determining if the specific trauma that would be treated by the EMDR was, in fact, neatly isolated, or, rather, something complicated and aggravated by a longer history of trauma. In part, the process was concerned with determining whether this was PTSD or *complex* PTSD.

As I answered his questions about my past and described various events – calmly and descriptively, as I felt neither shame nor pain except when discussing my daughter – I suspected him of being faintly astonished. His questions begat more questions, and I was surprised that by the end of our fourth session he was still compiling my "history", and we had not yet begun the EMDR. What might have seemed the simple isolation of one psychically undigested moment had become something much larger, complicated and diffuse.

Was my childhood in some diabolical concert with the incident? Hell, I didn't know.

—

Looking back now, the stages of my uncle's grooming were textbook. His behaviour was calculated to create a unique sense of trust and intimacy; a sense that nobody else understood me quite as well as he did.

He was staying with us from overseas. He first learnt my passions, which was not difficult given the musical and athletic objects of my worship were boldly declared by the posters on my bedroom wall. Then he ratified their importance.

Besides ingratiation, there was an additional tactical benefit for my uncle: it helped drive a wedge between me and my parents, who were inclined to believe my interest in sport frivolous and my musical taste decadent and antisocial. Forty years separate my father and me, and never will that distance seem as vast and unbridgeable as when I was a teenager playing punk or hip-hop in my bedroom.

These points of alienation – or mutual bafflement – between parents and their children are strategically important to the sexual predator. By insinuating himself into this space, and by flattering my tastes, my uncle shrewdly distinguished himself from my parents and offered himself as a hip confidant. "Rap has its own language," he would say. "As articulate as any other. It's a creative reclamation." In gratifying my interest in hip-hop, my uncle was also doing something more subtle – he was allying himself with me on a contentious domestic matter and thus generating the frisson of conspiracy. Developing a sense of conspiracy is important to the paedophile because it both flatters the victim and helps generate the conditions of secrecy. It was a beachhead – a landing ground from which further territory could be progressively claimed.

One night he asked me to play him the latest Oasis album, of which he knew I was enamoured. We were in my bedroom, and he asked that I turn off the lights. I thought this was strange and politely objected. But he insisted. He said the light of the stereo's LED display would be sufficient. I obliged, and the room went black. My uncle was a guest, and as discomforting as the darkness was, I was more concerned about being impolite.

It didn't occur to me that this was sinister – it seemed more likely to be an expression of my uncle's eccentricity.

Nothing more happened that night, except that my uncle rhapsodised about the genius of the Gallagher brothers. Which was part of his plan.

In the following week or so, he bought me beer and music. He told me he'd once met Roy Keane, then captain of Manchester United, and riffed philosophically on his temperament. He spoke in confounding ways about pop music and Irish nationalism, and by doing so implied his faith in my intelligence. He found ways to be physically close to me, like when he learnt that I cut mates' hair and asked for a trim. I agreed.

And while he was carefully eroding boundaries, and secretly replacing them with others, I naively saw a refreshing kind of bohemianism – an unusually relaxed and cultured man, a type of man I'd never known.

One day, he suggested that we go to the local pub, which sat beside a jetty on the nearby marina. This was another secret conscription and another transgression. My parents wouldn't have permitted this. Alcohol was strictly prohibited to their underage children, which he must have known.

Naturally, I was thrilled, and I asked my uncle if I could invite some friends. I was excited to show him off. He said no, offering an assortment of now forgotten reasons. Again, I deferred.

I wonder now what innocent excuses he'd prepared in case our pub journey was discovered. It was high-risk, after all: teens can't typically hold their booze. Maybe he had no excuses ready, but I'd bet that he did. I'd bet that he'd anticipated discovery. I'd bet that in his lifetime he'd pre-emptively written many excuses and alibis. In retrospect, he seemed practised. Assured in his methods.

It didn't go well for my uncle. I had barely touched my pint when I was spotted by a neighbour, who notified the manager that I was underage. We were asked to leave. Any novelty or excitement about being invited to a pub by an adult evaporated with the humiliation, and I wanted to go home. My uncle wouldn't have it. After all, he said, the pub had a takeaway bottle shop. I demurred; he insisted. He bought a six-pack, maybe two, and suggested we drink the beer on the rock wall of the harbour. And so we did.

I suppose my uncle would have preferred me cripplingly drunk. And I wonder what would have happened if I was. But my humiliation and creeping unease ensured that I drank very slowly that night, and I never got drunk. As I sipped from my tin, and he powered through them, my uncle revived his tactical flattery. Before the tiny, gentle waves of the harbour, he invited philosophical reflections from me and then applauded their acuity.

Tired and confused, I suggested, again, that we go home. We did. My uncle brought the remaining beer with him, and when we got to the side door he whispered that we should be quiet so that we didn't wake my parents. Then he suggested that he bring the beers to my room.

God, I was tired. And hard as this will be for many people to understand – and, trust me, I know just how difficult it is – I agreed. I felt some unease, but greater unease with the thought that I was badly misinterpreting my uncle. The fear of offending someone – of getting something so serious so wrong – was a vastly greater force than my judgement of the situation.

When he was on top of me, kissing my face, I felt the harshness of his whiskers, a sense of disgust, and profound confusion. And I remember telling myself two opposing things, over and over, in a fierce loop: This *still* isn't what it seems; and surely this can't be happening *again* (another story – I haven't been terribly lucky in this regard).

I experienced a kind of paralysis, so I'm unsure how I got my uncle out of my room. I don't remember. Then I said nothing. To anyone. And I should have. Because on another night, he'd return.

–

It's difficult writing about the next time. But I can lean upon one detail because, in my mind, it has become a synecdoche for the abuse. Earlier that evening, I'd gone with my family and uncle to a relative's house for dinner. They had cable TV, and while the adults were gathered round the dining table, I was pleased to find live coverage of the opening round of the English Premier League. It was Saturday, 16 August 1998. The broadcast fixture was Southampton at home to Liverpool. The Saints were in their typical red-and-white candy stripes; the Reds were debuting a garishly yellow away shirt.

There were signs that Liverpool remain defensively suspect, a problem uncorrected from previous seasons, and were especially vulnerable to Southampton's crosses into the box.

I think he'd drunk a lot that night. I remember smelling the booze on his breath. Maybe he required drink's blotting of conscience, its loosening of inhibition. Then again, his grooming was practised sober.

But the Reds, in a season they must privately hope can end their drought of league titles, possess a formidable midfield, and McAteer and McManaman were lively.

I think I slapped him. Did I slap him? How could I, when I was paralysed? And yet, there was some physical rebellion. I'm sure of it. Or am I? Is it that I just need to believe that I physically rebelled? Is that it? And has this need, over years, consolidated itself as a false memory?

Ince and Owen obliged fine saves early from Southampton 'keeper, Paul Jones. I remember him laughing when I hit him. Well, I think I hit him. Certainly, he laughed. I remember that. Why did he laugh? Was my slap, punch, wrestling so weak? Were my objections funny to him? *After a sluggish start, an increasingly confident home side went a goal up in the thirty-sixth minute when Norwegian national Egil Østenstad headed home after a right-side cross troubled the Liverpool defenders.* How amazing it is now to contemplate how infinitely elastic the benefit of my doubt was. *But within just two minutes, Liverpool had equalised when a lofted Michael Owen ball found the head of Karl-Heinz Riedle.*

Why didn't I fight more? I was big enough, old enough. *Southampton may feel cheated by the circumstances of Liverpool's second, match-winning goal. After a brutal collision with his own goalkeeper, the referee was concerned that full-back Jason Dodd was suffering from concussion and sent him from the field for inspection.*

I got him out of my room – or maybe he just left. Either way, I vowed never to tell anyone. I remember lying in the bath the next morning when I made this pledge. I remember staying in that bath for a long time, periodically refreshing the hot water, and staring at the rippled skin on my fingers. And I remember some of my thinking, which was stained with adolescent grandiosity: my parents had too much to think about as it was. I would save them some trouble.

The next night, I went to a party. I played spin the bottle and kissed a girl. Then I stayed the night at a friend's house because I couldn't bear returning home. The next day I made sure to stay out, and when I reluctantly but necessarily returned home late in the afternoon, my uncle was gone. My parents' discovery of what happened is another story. But Dad had packed my uncle's bags and driven him away.

My bed was irradiated, and I made my way back to it slowly, in stages. For the first forty-eight hours, I tried to avoid home. Then for the next week or so, I slept in front of the television in the family room. When I returned to my bedroom, I slept on its floor for a few weeks. Then, when I finally re-entered ground zero, I made sure to sleep with my head at the other end of the bed. Baby steps.

And none of this is the worst of what happened. But I can't write about the worst.

—

I was on medication now, which I thought was helping, after the few days of nausea and strange leg spasms had passed. But the more my therapist learnt, the more delayed the EMDR became. I thought it was all quite simple, but evidently it wasn't.

He was a gentle man, and I felt comfortable with him. But I also sensed that the discrete borders that work best with EMDR had now, via his excavations, been messily broadened.

So we changed its parameters, and he walked me through designing a tranquil mental space – an image, carefully detailed, that might be depended upon for comfort. I chose a lake in New Zealand I'd once kayaked on. Then there was the engineering of another mental object – a vault of sorts in which to securely store painful thoughts.

Finally, EMDR began. The idea is that traumatic memories are sometimes poorly stored – are not processed in such a manner that your mind accepts that the danger has passed. You don't discuss the traumatic moment during the therapy. Instead, the therapist sits closely in front of you and moves two raised fingers left and right, fairly quickly, and you follow them with your eyes while he asks you to silently summon the moment of the trauma while being attentive to both your emotional and somatic responses.

It felt like juggling, and I was painfully aware of thoughts that I assumed were of no use and, in fact, might be disastrously distracting me from the therapy's benefits. I thought that the therapist's arm must be really tired, and felt bad that I'd encouraged it. Then I thought that thinking such things was a waste of his time and mine, so I thought about returning to the moment but was aware of my effort in doing so.

And so on and so on. Silly, recursive loops. But there was no pain, other than the pain of thinking I was doing it all wrong – that my mind was simply too damn busy.

–

The years of Melbourne's Covid lockdowns are recalled with comfortable detachment and partial amnesia now, the strangeness reduced to a residue rather than vividly specific memories. Or they are until I read diary entries and abandoned pieces from that time – mostly about space exploration and its effects upon the minds of the explorers – and then a sense of the bizarre psychic humidity returns to me.

During one of the lockdowns, I had come across the story of Russian cosmonaut Oleg Skripochka, who, on his very first spacewalk in 2010, outside the International Space Station, became untethered. Drifting into space, he struck an antenna, then happily rebounded towards the station and a handhold. By an extraordinary fluke, he was safe.

I found this story in the memoir of NASA astronaut Scott Kelly, who was inside the station at the time. Little else can be found about the moment. Kelly wrote:

> I've often pondered what we would have done if we'd known he was drifting irretrievably away from the station. It probably

would have been possible to tie his family into the comm system in his spacesuit so they could say good-bye before the rising CO_2 or oxygen deprivation caused him to lose consciousness.

I couldn't stop thinking about this and wrote a short story inspired by it, probably the first short story I'd written since I was a teenager. The story was really about my daughter. It opened:

> Three years earlier, when his wife asked him why he had married and had a child with her, he answered by listing her virtues. They both knew this was dishonest. She had not asked what first attracted him – she was asking why he had bothered, when he had a greater commitment to the stars.
>
> He recalled this now, as he drifted, untethered. His cables had a two-failure tolerance. There had been three. He was gone now, "overboard" they called it, with almost four hours of oxygen left – enough time, maybe, for one orbit of Earth.

–

The treatment helped. It was the combination of talk therapy, EMDR and medication – as well as the surrendering of my own silence and the labour of maintaining a fairly successful, though lonely and exhausting, pretence of health.

But improvement is not linear, and it can be hard to judge. Convalescence isn't neatly progressive or as predictable as it might be for a broken arm, say, and I'm often unsure what to say when asked – by myself or by others – how I am. *Better*, I say, and I think that's right. But I'm frustrated by my inability to describe that improvement, or to have faith in its permanence.

—

This is just about the last you'll hear about me in this book, at least until the very end. There are three principal subjects of it, and I'm not one of them. In writing about them, I always reserved the right to introduce my own experiences where I thought they might complement something. But I didn't need to. It's enough, I think, for my experience to be largely contained here; how your knowledge of it informs what you read beyond this point will be determined by you.

What follows are the stories of three former emergency workers, each profoundly touched by trauma: a paramedic, a copper and a firie. Two of them have been diagnosed with severe PTSD. Tara, the firefighter, has not been. But childhood trauma both encouraged her to join the fire service and framed her experience of it.

You will, I think, learn much about their respective professions – but you will learn much more about the three people themselves. This book was never meant to be a general treatment of their jobs, nor a survey of trauma's literature as it applies to first responders. Such approaches might make for a more practical book, but they weren't the ones I chose. Instead, I wanted to intimately profile three human beings who defined themselves, for good or bad, by their vocations. All three had determined to find a career, not merely a job, and this distinction was about more than longevity. Each sought employment that they considered worthy – work that practically and unmistakably helped the public. Ultimately, each came to see their work as a central and inescapable part of their self-conception. For Brett and Tara especially, a career in emergency services provided a kind of emotional scaffolding: it helped them to defy sickly self-esteem and to define an otherwise uncertain sense of identity.

There were at least two problems with such emotional investment in their work, experienced by all three. The first is obvious: what happens when you leave the job? The short answer is a kind of existential crisis, made worse by the injuries you've acquired, which limit your ability to reinvent yourself. The second is the undermining of one's world view. All three subjects, like many first responders, had fairly blunt schemas for the world: by their own admission, they viewed things in black and white, and felt confident distinguishing between good and bad, right and wrong. Their professions initially fit into this world view: being an emergency worker was obviously a noble duty, an unalloyed public good. But when they encountered corruption, insensitivity or bureaucratic ineptitude, their comforting assumptions started to unwind.

I suppose that each of their stories could be read discretely, but some time ago I hoped that elements of their experiences might naturally chime with each other, without my co-ordination or contrivance. And so it was. Sometimes the chiming is faint and sometimes it's shrill, but it is unmistakably there.

This book began with a fairly narrow interest in PTSD and emergency work but grew to acquire a trio of themes. How did these people choose their professions? What did this kind of work do to them as individuals? And finally, I wanted to take an intimate look at the face of PTSD. These themes emerged naturally, through my many conversations with them.

Those three themes are the major ones, but there are others. Much time is spent, for instance, on their respective childhoods, two of which were distinctly and dramatically traumatic. One reason for this attention is to understand their work in a larger and more profound context. If the three subjects came to see themselves as being wholly defined by their work, I saw and was interested in much more about them. We may think of the work of first responders as something that can lead to clinical trauma, and it is. But in the case of these three, trauma also led them to their work. In different but arguably inexorable ways, their childhood trauma encouraged their work, and their work refracted their childhood experiences in complicated ways – and so this book swells and sighs with the bitter ironies that follow from such a relationship. The past is always present.

If this book does not focus exclusively upon their professional years, nor does it narrow itself to these three lives alone. You will also read about people who were consequential to each of them and, ultimately, to me: their family members, friends and colleagues, as well as others – including my grandfather – whose stories were seldom far from my mind as I wrote this book.

There is no shortage of hacky books about atrocities – works bloated with lurid descriptions of gunshot wounds and clotted with dates and times, the former for entertainment, and the latter to suggest authority. If their clichés don't numb you, their sustained indifference to psychology will. I've long felt that journalists have largely vacated the space of inner drama. Little attention, or little sophisticated attention, is paid to the contents of people's heads, even though they contain conflicts every bit as rich and interesting as "external" drama. In this book, you will read about the professional lives of emergency workers – murders, sieges, historic bushfires – but also about what happens in the *minds* of the people who respond to these crises.

All three impressed me with their candour and their willingness to reflect on all manner of things – fate, faith, regret and hope. They were both proud and self-deprecating, each remade by their work and by their injuries.

I don't know if they're heroes or not. I'm allergic to the word. I do know that they committed themselves to dangerous and necessary jobs, jobs heavy with physical, psychological and moral dangers. I wanted to know why and how they did those jobs and what those jobs did to them.

And they told me.

1

The Paramedic

PETER JAMES

"The difference between emergency service workers and the military is that we live in our war zone."

One of Peter's first jobs was driving to the midwifery home for single mothers on Monday mornings to collect the gauze-wrapped bodies of stillborn babies and place them in cardboard boxes once used to pack margarine. There was one baby per box, and on some days he would carry as many as seven or eight boxes to his ambulance. Then he would drive to the Royal Hobart Hospital's mortuary, where he would unload the boxes and place them carefully on the sandstone shelves of the mortuary's fridge. Once, he transferred miscarried triplets.

This job was called the "baby run". It was 1977, and Peter James was seventeen, a student paramedic. "Your brain takes a photograph every now and then," Peter told me, "and you can recall it as clearly as looking at a photo." These were his first photos of what would become thousands.

At the time he thought he was unaffected, but many years later, swept in on the tides of trauma after Peter became a father, those babies would revisit him. He would think about the insulting crudeness of their packaging, to which, in his naive and well-meaning deference, he was mostly oblivious at the time. He was also oblivious that this was his first moral injury, subtler than the later ones, but the first time that the virgin smoothness of his values – in this case, respect for the dead – met the coarseness of reality. Hospitals weren't churches but logistical sites, and death and disease had their processes. Forty years later, he would tell a senate inquiry: "At the time this did not impact me, but as the years and decades have rolled on, I think about this often."

Peter is a tall man; he still wears the moustache he first cultivated in the '70s, but he stoops slightly and shuffles now, his confidence and physical charisma long dissolved in the acid bath of trauma.

–

Peter was born in Manly, in Sydney's north, in 1959, the youngest of two. He was a shy and sensitive boy, bewildered by his parents' divorce when he was ten. "The world turns on its head," Peter said. "Your toys are boxed up, and you move schools."

He wondered if he was to blame, and for years hoped vainly for their reunion. This guilt and yearning were suppressed, and he never discussed the divorce with his parents. Today, both are gone, and he's still unsure of its causes.

It was an early lesson in the impermanence of things, something that decades later, after the massacre and the earthquakes, the suicides, domestic shootings, road wrecks and SIDS deaths, would resolve into a melancholic fixation: that families dissolve, buildings collapse and peace is broken.

After the divorce, Peter stayed with his grandmother and changed schools to Manly Primary. It was the only school he ever felt comfortable in. He can't really say why, but he recalls gentle teachers and the sound of cicadas outside the classroom in summer. Some mornings, on his way to school, he'd wander to the beach if the surf was up and sit and watch the breakers. His school was less than a hundred feet away, and when he heard its bell he stood, brushed the sand off his legs and trundled obediently to class.

He often fished with the boy next door, and sometimes rowed his tiny inflatable boat out onto the busy Sydney Harbour by himself, resting beside a navigation buoy and watching the larger boats go by.

Peter didn't know it at the time, but his great-grandfather had professionally fished these same waters, and while doing so had pulled many children, women and men from them. William Sly was one of five brothers, all of them locally renowned fishermen. The newspapers regularly reported the size of their catches and the details of their rescues.

On May 15, 1908, shortly before midnight, a man named James Davidson fell into the water from the passenger wharf, Manly. William Sly, who was on the wharf at the time, dived, fully dressed, into the water, and reaching Davidson held him up, at the same time calling out for assistance. His cries attracted the attention of Stanley Wild, who assisted Sly out of the water, and Davidson was got on to the wharf by means of the line which Sly had previously tied round him; but after prolonged efforts had been made by Dr. Hall and others to restore animation, life was pronounced extinct.

About six o'clock last evening a boy named R. White, residing in Cliff Street, Manly, fell into the water while fishing. A wharf-hand, W. Sly, who is employed at Manly, immediately jumped in, fully dressed, and rescued the boy, who was none the worse for his experience.

Florence Simpson, a domestic servant, aged 18, was charged before the Water Police Court yesterday with attempting to commit suicide by drowning herself. The evidence was that George Sly, a fisherman, was fishing off Blue Fish Point, at Manly, on Monday last, when he heard screams. He pulled in the direction of the sound, and saw a woman struggling in the breakers. With some difficulty he managed to rescue her from her dangerous position. She was then quite unconscious. Subsequently she was taken to the Manly Cottage Hospital, where she remained until yesterday. Constable Gippel went to the spot at which she was rescued, and later on charged her with attempting to commit

> suicide. She had gone over the rocks from a height of about 20ft. An hour's imprisonment was ordered by the Bench formally, and the girl was taken away by some friends.

One of the brothers found Henry Lawson at the bottom of Manly cliffs after a suicide attempt in 1902. In a brief newspaper column many years later, Frank Hardy wrote:

> Years after his fall from the cliff at Manly, Lawson revealed that a fisherman named Sly had rescued him from the rocks. Sly took him to Sydney Hospital. Lawson later told poet-friend Edward Brady that he was "Sly by name and sly by nature" because, when taking his leave of Henry at the hospital, Sly had said: "Better luck next time, Mr Lawson!"

In the land of the Sly brothers, suicide was illegal, an affront to nature. As was daytime swimming, so threatening were demiclad bathers to moral order. A year after Lawson's rescue, in 1903, the fifty-year-old prohibition on swimming was lifted in the Manly area, and the brothers established the Manly Surf and Life Saving Club, only the country's second. It was in these waters, more than a century later, that Peter scattered the ashes of his mother.

—

Peter's father worked at a plastics factory, and sometimes Peter helped there by grounding discarded goods for recycling or taking defective cassette tapes and separating their clear plastic from the dark. The air was warm and thick with the sweet fumes of plastic, and he was sufficiently diligent that his father's boss proposed to sponsor him for a scholarship at a plastics and chemical institute. But Peter had already decided: he wanted a career, not a job. He wanted to be a paramedic like his grandfather Eric Manly Gray.

He'd heard a few stories about his grandfather's work. How he had rescued children from an overturned bus. How hydrogen cyanide was once a common fumigant, and how frequently people were poisoned by it – including his grandfather, who collapsed in 1943 after entering a house to treat victims and was taken to hospital in his own ambulance.

Just before Christmas 1974, after meeting his son-in-law, Peter's father, for a few beers at the Manly Hotel, Peter's grandfather was bashed to death as he walked home. He was found in a laneway the next morning. He was sixty-seven. Police never found the killer. Peter was fifteen at the time and, as with the divorce, never spoke about the murder with his parents.

"He loved his cricket and a beer," Peter said of his grandfather. "I remember the cyanide wrecked his lungs, and he smoked heavily to stop the coughing for the rest of his life. His death knocked my father around. They were best mates. There was a big funeral, and I remember they played the hymn 'Rock of Ages'. He was buried, and his wife used to visit his grave every Sunday. I liked visiting, but I'd never get buried – I don't want to become a chore to others to visit and remember."

—

As a student paramedic, on the days that he wasn't on the road, transporting bodies or stretchers or tanks of oxygen, Peter was assigned to the dispatch centre, where he answered the public's emergency calls. There was little instruction, just a quick demonstration of the switchboard, and he was often left alone in the ambulance station. Nearby was an aluminium coffin reserved for decomposed bodies; when trucks drove by, the coffin rattled noisily with the vibrations.

"I don't remember being nervous," Peter said. "I just got on with it. There was a lot of trust, and there were no stuff-ups, but I wouldn't dream of letting a seventeen-year-old take the calls today."

In those days, in the late '70s and early '80s, there were three shifts: 8 a.m. to 4 p.m, 4 p.m. to midnight, and midnight to 8 a.m. If you finished at midnight you'd head to the casino for beers, or across the road to the carpark of a petrol station with slabs of your own. In the middle of the carpark was a half 44-gallon drum, stuffed with wood. The paramedics and coppers would gather round the fire with their cans of beer, sometimes sitting on the bonnets of the police cars, their engines still running to keep their arses warm in the winter. They were exclusively male, and they would shoot the breeze and stoke the fire and transform their arcane knowledge of death and transgression into pitch-black banter.

One night, when the wood ran low, a few of the coppers walked over to a nearby property occupied by some well-known "dropkicks" who'd too often demanded their attention. The police kicked the fence down, broke up the planks with their boots and brought the wood back to the fire.

"We didn't have deep and meaningful discussions then," Peter said. "Black humour was a big thing, a vent for us. We were unwinding but not realising it. Drinking became the norm. The term PTSD didn't exist, but we were always coming across someone who was having the first day, or last day, or worst day of their life."

And Peter loved it, even later when it broke him.

—

They were in Scotland, the second stop of their honeymoon, and Peter remembers the discomfort of wearing heavy clothes on sunburnt skin. From Hawaii they had come to visit Christine's grandparents in the old coal mining town of Cardenden near the Fife coast, where it was quiet and windy and grey.

It was the first week of May 1986. Peter was twenty-six, his new wife Christine twenty-one, and 3300 kilometres away the ruptured No. 4 reactor of the Chernobyl nuclear plant was issuing a radioactive cloud across Europe. You couldn't see the radiation, but if the winds were right and there was heavy rainfall, the rain would carry radionuclides to the earth. In Cardenden, newsmen on the radio warned against going outside if it was raining. There was a sharp increase in sales of bottled water, and commensurate declines in sales of milk. Farmers bought Geiger counters and slaughtered their livestock. Across Britain, thousands of cows, sheep and chickens were culled.

Peter said to Christine: "It's following us." He wasn't referring to the radiation, but to the powerful sense that strange calamities seemed to stick to them "like shit to a blanket". From Scotland, they drove south to England's Lake District. They stayed near Ambleside, a small town at the top of England's largest natural lake, half an hour's walk from Rydal Mount, where William Wordsworth lived for almost forty years before his death.

Wordsworth returned to the district in 1799, after a short trip to Germany left him homesick, and began to consecrate the area's beauty in poetry. *Of majesty, and beauty, and repose, / A blended holiness of earth and sky.* In 1818, the younger poet John Keats made a pilgrimage to Rydal Mount, and from the road he wrote to his brother in London:

> We walked here to Ambleside yesterday along the border of Windermere, all beautiful with wooded shores and islands. Our road was a winding lane, wooded on each side, and green overhead, full of foxgloves – every now and then a glimpse of the lake, and all the while Kirkstone and other large hills nestled together in a sort of grey black mist …
>
> I shall learn poetry here and shall henceforth write, more than ever, for the abstract endeavour of being able to add a mite to that mass of beauty which is harvested from these grand materials, by the finest spirits, and put into ethereal existence for the relish of one's fellows. I cannot think with Hazlitt that these scenes make man appear little. I never forgot my stature so completely; I live in the eye, and my imagination, surpassed, is at rest.

Keats never met Wordsworth. The elder poet was out campaigning for the re-election of one of his wealthy patrons when

Keats arrived. The blistered poet left a note. But Wordsworth would have approved of Keats's letter, the one describing the blissful surrender of his imagination. In his poetry, Wordsworth encouraged his readers to acquire a meditative passiveness amid nature, as so the mind emptied itself of conscious agitations and *just was*.

Therapists would later tutor Peter in meditation, encouraging a similar state. Sometimes, with a sunny deck and the companionship of his cat, he could achieve it. But not often, and not for long. The memories were too intrusive. Radionuclides falling to earth.

—

As Chernobyl invisibly contaminated Europe, Peter and Christine walked the mossy trails around Windermere Lake. Local farmers were destroying their milk and slaughtering their animals.

"I think creating order out of bloody chaos was one of the big reasons I became a paramedic," Peter said. "I'm black and white when it comes to a lot of stuff, and if it's broken, it needs fixing."

But the problem with wanting to impose order upon chaos is that chaos is perpetually generated. Nuclear reactors ignite, parents split, laneways are fatefully chosen. Peter wonders if his need to impose order originated in his parents' divorce. He can't say for sure, but there is some psychological research suggesting a link between a pre-existing intolerance for uncertainty and a higher susceptibility to post-traumatic stress symptoms. "One psychological vulnerability factor that may convey risk for increased PTSS is Intolerance of Uncertainty (IU)," a 2016 paper in the *Journal of Anxiety Disorders* reads. "Individuals high in IU display a tendency to respond negatively to uncertain or ambiguous situations on a cognitive, emotional, and behavioural level."

When the couple returned to Scotland two years later, Pan Am Flight 103 was blown up while flying over the town of Lockerbie. All 259 passengers and crew died – as did another eleven people on the ground, when large parts of the aircraft fell across a residential street.

It was upon this world that Peter wanted to impose order. It was this world whose wounds he wanted to staunch.

–

Uncertainty is unavoidable in emergency work, and first responders often find themselves in violently unpredictable situations. How they are supported in the aftermath can determine the emotional impact of such events. I spoke about this with Mike Ryan, a clinical psychologist who joined the Tasmania Police in 1995. He helped to recruit cadets, advised police negotiators and counselled officers. When we met, some years ago now, he had recently retired and was rediscovering archery – "an elegant and meditational sport", he told me. "And you can only attribute the quality of your shot to yourself. If the definition of maturity is taking responsibility for your actions, then archery teaches that."

Ryan explained his model for predicting and evaluating the emotional impact of events upon police. "It's not an original of mine," he said. "I got it off a colleague about twenty years ago." The model breaks challenging situations down into three parts: demand, control and predictability. When training police, Ryan used an old episode of British police drama *The Bill* to illustrate it. The episode is called "FAT'AC" – police shorthand for "fatal accident" – and it opens with genial beat cop Yorkie patrolling his patch of London. He's calm, contented and in control. He stops to admire a parked Ferrari, then smiles as a mother pushes her child by in a pram. The sun is shining, and the viewer is impressed with Yorkie's sense of peace and community.

And then: the sound of squealing tyres, smashed metal and a jammed car horn. The idyll is broken.

"He's not prepared for anything," Ryan said. "Suddenly there's a screech of brakes and he turns around and sees a car with an elderly lady, and a mother and baby have gone under a truck. The mother and baby are decapitated. The old woman is lying on the road, injured. So he goes from zero … to bang! The level of demand is very high. Like any good cop, he radios for backup. And they say, 'We can't give you backup because there's a fire and the roads are blocked. Deal with it.' So, you can see his control diminish. The driver's drunk and tries to get out of the car. A witness tries to fight the driver. Yorkie sees the decapitated mother and baby. A woman is bleeding to death. He forgets to take notes. Using my model, there's low control, high demand and low predictability."

Yorkie, forgivably, makes a mess of things. He's overwhelmed by the cascading chaos, and without support there is a desperate triaging of priorities. He writes unusable notes and lets witnesses leave before he has taken statements. But when Ryan showed this episode to police, he wasn't just asking them to consider Yorkie's actions. He was also asking senior officers to ask better questions of their staff during debriefs.

"When Yorkie finally gets back to the station, the sergeant says, 'You really cocked that up, didn't you? You didn't take notes. You let witnesses get away.' Yorkie goes into the crib room to have a meal and sits by himself, and someone says, 'What's wrong with Yorkie?' and they respond, 'Oh, just a FAT'AC.' So they look at the content, but they don't look at his experience. But then the good sergeant calls him over and asks 'What happened?' and lets him talk about it.

"We use that in training, and we ask: 'Which sergeant do you want to be?' Because what buffers this stress – the high demand, low control, low predictability – is the level of personal support and value [you receive]. Coppers are a very insular group, so it's important to get support from your colleagues. Being told your experience was okay by another police officer is very important."

There are two things to note here. First, that extreme stress and witnessing the grotesque do not guarantee trauma, and preparedness for it lessens the odds of acquiring it. "Motor vehicle accidents are less traumatic than people think because they're predictable," Ryan said. "Coppers have a fair idea of what they'll encounter. Might be bodies decapitated, bodies flayed going through a windscreen – it might be awful. But it's predictable. They close off the area, they get witness statements. They have a preparedness. But with domestics, it could be anything."

Ryan told me the story of a friend, a police officer, who was called to a domestic dispute after neighbours complained about noise. With his partner, he arrived expecting the situation to be low demand, high control and low predictability. But when the door was opened, and a shotgun was levelled at his head, it suddenly became a "fucking lot of demand, no control and huge unpredictability".

The second thing is the importance of senior officers asking the right questions of their staff, ones that might liberate them from shame or embarrassment. This isn't just a matter of empathy or sensitivity; it's a question of whether senior officers have the time, patience and interest to act upon what they've heard. If they don't, sometimes it's easier to ask the deliberately narrowing question, or none at all.

"I had one client who was part of some officers called to a melee at a mall," Ryan said. "They go down there, and this officer gets involved and suddenly slips over. He doesn't have his gun properly secured, so he loses his Glock. He's on the ground, and he told me later that in an instant he thought, 'I'm gonna die. I'm gonna be killed.'

"Within a few seconds he regains his gun, gets back on his feet, sorts a few people out – perhaps a little more vigorously than he should have. But that microsecond of thinking he was going to die, that's what stayed with him. And he couldn't understand it … Police are results-oriented. He goes back to the station, and the sergeant says, 'Good job: you arrested the guys, good result.' But this chap was thinking – and he couldn't say it to anyone – that he could have died. Good sergeants, they ask:

'Tell me what happened', not 'How do you feel?', because then you get more of the story."

I thought of all of this again when Peter James told me the Lebrina story.

The call was simple, but unnervingly light on detail: a gunshot had been reported by a neighbour. That's all they had. That and the address: a modest weatherboard home in Lebrina, a small, depressed town half an hour's drive from Launceston. Peter and his colleague flicked the lights and sirens. They arrived before the police. It was 28 July 1993.

Peter knew how volatile and dangerous domestic calls could be. He'd once arrived at a home where a man had been stabbed. Peter was alone – the police weren't there yet. "It was just me, the patient and the bloke who stabbed him," Peter remembers. "And all you can do is ask permission. So, I asked: 'Can I treat him?' and he goes, 'Yeah.' And knowing he's said 'yes', you know you're safe, but if he says 'no' then you just wait for the police."

Peter and his colleague entered the Lebrina home, and there he was: a man graphically deceased on the couch in the front room, his shotgun beside him. The house was silent. Peter started packing up their gear, while his colleague checked the other rooms. There was a bright spray of blood on the bathroom mirror, where they assumed the man had first attempted to kill himself. Then Peter's colleague opened the bedroom door and found them: the man's young wife and toddler daughter, slumped in a corner, each with a single .22 bullet wound in their head. Both were unconscious but still shallowly breathing.

"So we go from an operational mode to wind-down mode and putting our gear away, to suddenly back up to bloody full operational mode," Peter said. "I felt like I was moving in slow motion. I scooped the baby up, and on the way out of the house I kicked the chest of the guy. I don't remember that part. Obviously, it was anger, but I've no recollection of it. I was told about it later.

"What I do remember, clear as a bell, is being in the ambulance with the baby. My colleague had taken the wife into another ambulance. And once we started ventilating the baby, there was brain matter coming out of the [bullet] hole, which indicates that the bullet had gone through the base of the skull as well. But the mother and baby were [going to be] used for organ donations, so I was in the resus seat still doing resus, because if I hadn't resuscitated the baby, the organs would have been wasted. You're trying to do the best you can with what you have in front of you. From what I gather from the others, I was pretty uptight."

Peter has kept the case notes for very few calls. In fact, he thinks he only has two. One of them is Lebrina. "Some things you want to forget, but you hang onto," he said. His colleague wrote them in the hospital upon arrival. A small excerpt: "Evidence of brain matter – both entry & exit wounds and sock – r. foot + blood. Minimal blood loss from wounds."

"That one knocked me around," Peter said. "That started the downward spiral. Then twelve months later, Port Arthur happened."

In fact, the Port Arthur massacre happened three years later, but memory is fallible. After I find the Lebrina story in newspaper archives, which otherwise corroborate Peter's telling (as do the case notes and Peter's therapist at the time), I apologetically mention the discrepancy. He's surprised and concedes that the graphic obscenity of each event may have compressed their proximity in his mind. The murder of children in both cases, and the similarity in ages of those children to his own, have braided them together.

"That incident is always at the front of my mind," Simon Webb told me. Webb was a clinical psychologist who often worked with emergency personnel. At the time he was the Tasmanian Police psychologist – Mike Ryan's predecessor – and he met with Peter and his colleague after Lebrina in his capacity as head psychologist of the state's critical incident stress debriefing team. He has stayed in touch with Peter since his retirement. "I remember Peter's colleagues saying that Peter just grabbed the baby and went. And he had young kids too. Knowing that the woman and child had some vital signs, but were really gone ...

"That sort of thing happens too often. Too often. I did so many debriefs around that time. I did 367 debriefs [with emergency personnel] in one year. I'd be in a car at 3 o'clock in the morning, driving from the fucking west coast of Tasmania after doing debriefs, with cops or ambos with me. It was just constant for a few years there. You name it: shootings, stabbings, fires. Just incredible."

I asked Simon about Peter kicking the corpse as he left: if he knew about it at the time, if it was clinically significant, and if it signified something beyond a natural, instinctive contempt.

"It shows anger, but it might be a relatively normal reaction during an abnormal event," Simon said. "Management would have said it's unacceptable and made a big thing of it if they knew – I think some managers might forget what it's like when they were operating at the front. People are expected to go out and do these things over and over and over again, and be able to go home and sleep and not worry about it."

Peter did go home and fitfully tried to sleep. Before he went to bed, he kissed his two sons. One was three years old, the other eighteen months – the same age as the victim he'd cradled and desperately blown oxygen into that day.

He didn't tell his wife much. He rarely did. Peter tried to shield her. But it was a devil's bargain. His "protection" was painful for her. By withholding details, he became distant. Aloof. And Christine wasn't stupid. She knew when things were wrong. Peter assumed that he could neatly quarantine his experiences at work, but he couldn't. "Everybody knows there is no fineness or accuracy of suppression; if you hold down one thing you hold down the adjoining," Saul Bellow wrote. In trying to protect his wife, Peter engineered his emotional distance from her.

"In my experience, those who broke down were the ones who'd been on the frontline a very long time," Simon Webb said. "They were the ones who were always there. Who always said 'yes'. The ones who drove the fastest to scenes. The ones who pushed to the front of the pub brawl. The ones who were most committed. Sometimes to a fault, I guess. And I think Peter was one of them. Very well respected and totally committed. But he couldn't say no."

—

Simon Webb understood trauma intimately. He'd had a varied life before becoming a clinical psychologist: bright, prickly and unrooted, Webb was a high-school dropout, abattoir worker, shelf stacker and soldier all before his twentieth birthday. He joined the Australian Army in 1967, when he was eighteen; the next year he was sent on his first tour of Vietnam – a war he didn't much understand at the time, but which he was determined to understand after he returned badly damaged.

On 12 May 1968, about 20 kilometres north of Biên Hòa City, Australian troops established a fire support base they called Coral on an approach to Saigon. The area contained infiltration routes used by the Viet Cong in their attack on the South Vietnamese capital a week earlier, and the Australians wanted to surprise them on their withdrawal from the city, when they would presumably come back along the same tracks.

But the Australians had underestimated the size of the opposing forces, and their establishment of the base was "confused and protracted", in the words of historian Ashley Ekins. Viet Cong reconnaissance troops saw it, reported back and soon, quietly and under cover of darkness, began surrounding Coral. Before dawn on 13 May, the Viet Cong unleashed a heavy mortar and rocket attack on the base. Eleven Australian troops died; twenty-eight were wounded.

Simon Webb was one of the injured. A mortar shell exploded nearby, rupturing his eardrum and shredding his lower body with shrapnel. Later, on a giant Hercules plane, Webb was flown back to Australia with the other seriously wounded soldiers. His family met him at the airport. Webb was limping and yellowed from jaundice, and he can recall their shocked faces. What might have been a simple and joyous reunion was complicated by how alien his experience was, and how old emotional distances within the family were pronounced by it.

After this brief airport reunion, Webb was taken by an army ambulance to a military hospital in Brisbane. He stayed for a fortnight, and upon his discharge (his injuries were sufficiently serious that he would be periodically readmitted over the next six months), a taxi was called for him. "The driver just wanted to talk about the price of petrol, or who won the football," Webb remembers. "And I'm thinking to myself: '*Jesus*, mate, I've just come out of a war zone, what the fuck are you talking about?' People didn't really appreciate where I'd come from. But that's not their fault, that's just life."

An intense and complicated anger flourished after that. "Some of my anger, I think, was also tied up with my guilt and my shame about not being able to go back to my battalion," Webb said. "A feeling that I've deserted my mates. I spoke to other blokes who got wounded or shipped home early, and many of them had similar sorts of feelings."

The anger flourished, as did Webb's desire to better understand the war that had fatally mutilated his friends and asked him to do the same to others. But this only intensified his anger and sense of estrangement, because the more he read, the surer he was that the war was unjustified.

Webb told me that since he was a boy, he had often not known where he fit in. But after his return from Vietnam, this estrangement seemed especially acute: he was surrounded by civilians for whom his experiences were largely alien, uncommunicable and morally suspect; while in the army, he was mostly surrounded by people who earnestly believed the war was justified.

"I started going to the library when I was in and out of the hospital and getting everything I could find about the history of Vietnam, and their previous history with the French and Chinese," Webb told me. "And the more I read, the angrier I got. I read one book called *From Yalta to Vietnam*, which probably stirred me more than anything. I guess I've always been a little bit of a lefty, unlike members of my family who never could understand why I was like that. Anyway, I carried a lot of anger for quite some time. And the more I read, the more I realised that the whole war was bullshit."

Webb was clinically traumatised, but it took a very long time for him to realise it. He said PTSD "crept up on him", but another way of putting it might be that his *realisation* of his disorder finally caught up – as did modern psychology, which by the late 1970s was finally resolving the question of whether trauma was diagnosable.

Webb's trauma added to his anger, as did his isolation, his sense of shame about abandoning his mates, and the moral injury that follows from objecting to a war you have participated in. But there were symptoms other than rage. There was the drinking, the nightmares, the intrusive memories, and "for a long time, I was actually hearing what I think was a flashback of the mortar going off, the mortar that got me," Webb said. "I'd been at Mum and Dad's place once, and I heard this enormous *bang!* And I looked out to see what it was, and everyone else was going about their business – *it was all in my head*. That probably happened for ten years, or so. Auditory flashbacks, I think they called it."

There was a moment – a specific moment – when Webb realised he wasn't okay, and it was more than a decade after the Battle of Coral-Balmoral. It was early 1979, and he was now studying for his psychology degree at nights while working in the day as an army recruitment officer. He wasn't seeing much of his wife, and she suggested a date night to redress their distance. They should see a film, she said, and he agreed – although he never asked her what the film was.

It was *The Deer Hunter*, a graphic, controversial and multi-Oscar-winning feature about three Pennsylvanian steelworker mates conscripted to Vietnam. The film features gruesome battles, nightmarish sadism and the friends' bleakly tortured re-integration back home.

"I remember at the end of the movie, [my wife] said, 'We can go now,' and people were leaving," Webb said. "And I just sat there, couldn't move, just holding everything in, until just about everyone had left, and then I walked out and walked back to the car. I got into the car and burst into sobs. Just cried for about two hours, while my wife sat beside me until I sort of got a grip again. That's when I started realising there was an issue."

As he had done after his return from the war, Webb started hitting his university's library – this time to understand the war's mental effect upon him. There was an emerging psychological literature on war trauma, one that derived from the hundreds of thousands of returned US soldiers from Vietnam, and the next year, in 1980, "PTSD" first appeared in *The Diagnostic and Statistical Manual of Mental Disorders*.

Simon's career provided him with a substantial purpose, and his personal experiences enhanced his rapport with clients. But to treat traumatised veterans and emergency workers while experiencing PTSD yourself is to hold your hand very close to the flame. Over his career, Simon worked for veteran organisations, police forces and in private practice. He worked with the Port Arthur community after the massacre and volunteered his time as a mediator, liaising between traumatised people and the government departments he felt were insufficiently responsive.

"I guess I knew it was getting unhealthy in a way," Webb said. "It was put to me a few times by therapists that I've seen myself, that I've worked my butt off basically, so that I might end up seeing eight or nine people a day and spend weekends writing reports. I think trying to help people sort out their own stuff is one of the things we use to try and stop looking at our own."

His hearing gradually worsened too, a legacy of the mortar shell, and he began to realise a few years back that it could alarmingly warp communication with his patients. Mishearing can acquire heavy significance in therapy, and Simon realised he should call it a day. He has settled in Westbury, a small town just out of Launceston, and finally found a congenial RSL club – he had avoided them for many years because of their "cliquishness". After three failed marriages – casualties, he said, of his own poor instincts – he has "managed" to stay single for the past two decades. These days, it's just him, his books and his dog – and the odd schooner down at the local RSL. He still checks in with Peter, and one thing they share is Port Arthur.

–

When Martin Bryant drove his yellow Volvo to Port Arthur's historic site, its boot stuffed with high-powered and casually acquired weapons, Peter was living in Launceston. It was 28 April 1996.

Peter was on holiday at the time, but when he heard sketchy reports of a shooting on the radio, he called the critical incident stress debriefing team, where Simon Webb worked, to ask if he was needed. He was – not as a paramedic, but as a debriefer.

With two colleagues, Peter drove to Hobart, just over two hours away, where he was briefed at ambulance headquarters. Even there, he said, he doesn't remember the scale of the crimes being evident yet. He wasn't "steeling himself", he told me, as he drove to the police command post that had been established at a Tasmanian devil sanctuary in Taranna, about forty-five minutes from Hobart and close to Port Arthur.

Peter arrived at the command post sometime after 5 p.m., and police began explaining the scale of the slaughter. The number of deaths wasn't confirmed yet, they said, but it was unthinkably high, and the police and SES volunteers were now searching for survivors who may have crawled into bushland to hide. They also sketched for Peter the back routes to the historic site, because driving the most direct way would take him past the Seascape guesthouse, where Bryant was holed up and shooting at police.

When Peter arrived at Port Arthur, “the living had all been removed” and taken to hospitals. Rather than treat the physically wounded, Peter was there to support the volunteer ambulance service who were first on the scene – “people needed to ventilate, and it was my job to listen” – but he would quickly be asked to do much more. Peter would work at the site for almost twenty-four hours straight.

“I knew most of the senior police there,” he said, “because they’d been members of the critical incident debriefing team. After I’d done my debriefings, the police said, ‘You’re not going anywhere. We’ve got crime scene walkthroughs to do, and you’re gonna help us.’ And so I did. As graphic and disturbing as the place was, it was still a very large and complex crime scene, and there are logistics that go with that. Bodies had to be identified, and then forensic teams would go through again to examine the scene and photograph the bodies in position. I helped with that. I remember Tasmanian devils were starting to come out and sniff around the bodies, and the bodies had to be protected. Afterwards, they had to be loaded carefully and compassionately. These were all things that needed to be done. Forensics had so much to do.

“I would offer advice – try to reduce police fatigue by asking that they rotate the officers who were protecting bodies. A whole busload of police came after that to help. The cops were good, very responsive to my suggestions. I was also there to support people, as some were falling apart. For some who had seen the children, they had reminded them of their own. There were definitely a few who weren't doing so well, and I would become one of them the next day.

"There's black humour sometimes at jobs. But we operate behind a facade, and the magnitude of this, well, the facade fell away. And also when people become fatigued, like they did that day, coping mechanisms fall away."

The forensic processing of the scene, as well as the psychological triaging, went on through the night, all while Bryant was still holed up at the Seascape. He was largely surrounded, but as night fell there was no guarantee he couldn't slip away in the darkness. Those working at Port Arthur were on edge, and soon rumours were circulating that Bryant had indeed left the bed and breakfast and was returning to the site.

"It was a well-controlled scene," Peter said. "But we were all anxious. I remember going to the toilet, and hearing the crunching of footsteps outside, and thinking 'I don't want to die falling face first into a urinal.' I think it was the police commander.

"It was a dark, cold night. And it sucked the life out of you."

—

If there's a hell, Peter said, it would look like the Broad Arrow Café that day. It was in there, and the adjacent gift shop, that Bryant, in just ninety seconds, had fired twenty-nine rounds of his AR-15, killing twenty people and injuring another twelve.

When Peter approached the café to assist in the scene's processing, there was a police officer on guard at the front, signing in those who entered. He had a warning: "Just know that the man who goes in there will not be the same man who comes out," he said.

"Never has a truer word been spoken," said Peter.

When Peter stepped inside, he felt a familiar sensation – or a familiar absence of sensation. Everything felt magically still, silent. He couldn't feel his breath, or the turbulence of the ceiling fans that were still spinning. There were forensic officers, but he couldn't hear them speak – or at least, in his traumatically embalmed memory of the scene, there were no voices.

He was operating on another plane – some senses were hyperfocused and others numbed – and he remembers that room now as if it were a literal vacuum, sucked of air.

"I still can't eat potato wedges," Peter said. "Every second person had them hanging out of their mouth. The high-velocity bullets he used, they cause small entry wounds but massive exit wounds, and people had either their face completely gone or the back of their head completely gone. The images are clear as a bell.

"And no, don't worry about asking me about that day," Peter said. "As I've told my wife many times, you can't put anything into my head that's not already there."

I've thought a lot about the police guard's words to Peter, which were forgivably raw and honestly forbidding, but perhaps helped prime Peter for a grotesquely transformative experience. I am reminded of Mike Ryan's experience of the scene the following day. As Tasmania Police's chief psychologist, Ryan had spent the night attempting to make contact with Bryant in the Seascape, where it was believed he was holding its two owners hostage. The next morning, the commanding police officer asked Ryan to join the state's coroner at Port Arthur to help counsel "a few people who weren't doing so well".

"I found myself in Broad Arrow," Ryan told me. "And that didn't affect me at all. I'd never seen a dead body in my life, but I found it almost like a film set. I objectified it. [My response] was very interesting. I saw one body sitting up, looking like she was puzzling over something.

"I was waiting to be affected. The images stay with me. They're graphic. I'm not saying I was unaffected. One thing that really stays with me, and this is bizarre, but five of us were crammed into this little car, and it was the most perfect morning in Port Arthur, just the most beautiful, bizarre setting for this horrific institution. There were these mushrooms, red with white flakes on top – a whole row of them against this green swathe of grass. The sun was coming over. We just looked at it and said, 'It's so beautiful.' But there's two kids up there dead, and others lying around. Dead. The coroner said something like: 'You know, I'll never come back here again.' I've never been back, either."

—

Ryan explained to me how a hardened officer, who has previously detached themselves from the traumas they were called to, might suddenly – and profoundly – be affected when the event was personalised. He told me of an experienced police officer – "you could cut your hair on his chin" – who had come to see him after attending a fatal road accident.

The victim was a young girl – the same age as the police officer's daughter and wearing the same-coloured dress as she had been that morning when he said goodbye. "He told me it was just like getting shot," Ryan said. "He said, 'I dealt with it, did really well', but he [later] collapsed, and then it brought everything else back [from his career]. It still gives me goosebumps."

The same was true of Peter at Port Arthur, as it was for many others. As he was debriefing officers, conducting crime scene walkthroughs, arranging rosters and helping with the carriage of bodies, he was thinking of his own children, who were the same ages – six and three – as Alannah and Madeline Mikac, who were killed with their mother, Nanette. "It personalises it big time," Peter said. "Your brain sort of twists it, and I remember saying later to my wife, 'How could someone shoot Sam and Oliver?'"

Peter worked through the night – there was an interrupted half hour of sleep in a police van – and made a mutual agreement with a colleague: they would each call the other's wife, to let them know they were okay. "We were both so fatigued and emotional, we weren't up to talking to our spouses."

The next day, after news came that Bryant had been arrested, Peter was in a makeshift office at the site. The phone rang. "It was a tour operator, and he said, 'When's the place opening up? Because I've got tours booked,' and I said, 'Go and get fucked' and hung up."

Then the phone rang again. It was the producer of a commercial TV news program, asking Peter if he could speak live in a few hours. Peter murmured agreement, insincerely, then hung up. "I dunno who was gonna pick up the phone [when the producer called back], but it wasn't going to be me."

Peter's work wasn't done. He was sent to the Seascape guesthouse, where Bryant had held siege for twenty hours before torching it that morning; it was now a smoking ruin. On the small bridge over the creek to the property, Peter saw a senior police officer he knew. Standing nearby were two young men. They were the children of Seascape's owners, who had been Bryant's first victims the day before, although police had at first believed Bryant had held them hostage throughout the night. The police officer asked Peter to tell the young men that their parents were dead. "That was something I'd done many times before," Peter said. "Notifying someone of a death. I think they already knew, but you expect the worst and hope for the best."

Around 3 p.m. that afternoon, almost twenty-four hours after he had arrived, Peter called time. Some police officers wanted him to stay on, and Peter wasn't a man to say no, but his exhaustion and horror had peaked overwhelmingly. He wanted to get home. "I just couldn't go on," he said. "There's only so much you can tolerate."

So, Peter was driven home. It was a three-and-a-half-hour drive. He cried when he arrived. Hugged his wife and boys. But he didn't say much. And his house, if it wasn't before, became a castle. "My front door was like a drawbridge," Peter said. "I shut that door, and [the world] stayed outside."

While he was working at the massacre site, Peter had felt shame. There were different sources of his shame, some of them mysterious. There was the shame of being alive when children were dead, and shame that there was no one left to save. There was the subtler shame of witnessing a human's capacity for evil. And later, there was the stranger shame – or gross bewilderment – found in contemplating the abyss between the carnage and the perpetrator, who was proud and excited and smilingly oblivious of the infinitude of suffering he'd caused.

And maybe, although Peter doesn't say this, there was shame that he had closed the drawbridge to his own family. "I always wanted to protect my kids from some of the stuff I'd seen and done," he said. "But maybe I cut myself off too much."

—

Peter met Christine on a blind date in a Hobart pub. It was 1983. Although shy and without much experience of young women, the result of attending an all-boys high school, he was comfortable enough to finish her plate of chips. A good sign, he thought.

They started dating, and soon Peter declared that he thought they'd get married one day. They wed two years later.

"He was really easy to talk to," Christine remembered. "A really kind guy and genuine. He didn't have any airs or graces. I was a student nurse then, doing night duty when we started dating, and we'd do seven-night weeks. My mum said he'd seen me at my worst and was still coming around. I couldn't have asked for someone kinder than Peter. I got lucky and I still think that, even if things have been hard sometimes."

Christine gave birth to their first child, Sam, in the winter of 1990, the night Martina Navratilova won her ninth singles title at Wimbledon. Peter remembers that, as he remembers the storm and the leaking roof in the labour room, and the words he kept repeating to himself when presented with his son – "I'm a dad" – which echoed richly inside him. "He looked like a spider – he had arms and legs going everywhere – and it hit me: I'm a dad. I was amazed."

Peter and Christine had their second child, Oliver, two years later. By this time, they had moved to Launceston; it was a year before the Lebrina incident. "I certainly became more protective of my kids over the years," Peter said. "When we moved into this house in Launceston here, there was a swimming pool, and it was an above-ground one, but the top part was not even knee-high – just the perfect height for a toddler to topple into and drown – so I had the bloody thing ripped out and turned into a garden. I've been to the drownings of kids. I was aware of the safety things, but not to the point of – I mean, they rode bikes. I tried to work behind the scenes.

"It would be interesting, I guess, to know what they saw. Their perspective will be different. I remember, not too long after September 11, we went for a holiday to New Zealand as a family. And we went up into the Sky Tower in Auckland. And they've got these big thick glass panels that you look straight down on, and the two boys are jumping up and down, and it just freaked me out. I was sweating like a pig and white as a ghost. I was absolutely a wreck."

He pauses. "Over the years, the deaths of kids affected me more," he said. "It seemed such a waste of humanity."

—

After Port Arthur, Christine watched Peter fall into a severe depression, and in the months, then years, after the massacre, she became familiar with a song that Peter played "over and over and over again". It was "Ashokan Farewell", an instrumental lament written by American folk musician Jay Ungar in 1982, but which sounded as if it were written more than a century before. The documentary maker Ken Burns was fond of it and used it as the theme to his famous series on the American Civil War, which was where Peter first heard it.

"The song takes your brain on a walk," Peter said. "Port Arthur was a beautiful place, though I'll never want to see it again, and listening to that song, it's almost like you're strolling through the rose gardens there, which were beautiful. I'd been for picnics before the massacre. [The song] made you sad but lifted you up at the same time."

The song was also an unmistakable sign to Christine that her husband was "heading downhill again". Christine was working as a psych nurse, and the mother of two young boys, and they weren't wealthy – she worried about her husband, her children and herself. Peter was withdrawn, often unresponsive, and without support she wondered how she could raise two kids, repay the mortgage and maintain a compassionate poise while juggling intense responsibilities.

In this unforgiving context, Christine said something she later regretted. "I remember saying to him, 'Peter, you really need to – not get over this, but sort of get back on the straight and narrow, because you have kids and your work,'" Christine told me. "I feel really bad that I said it. I probably just said it flippantly. And I think it was really belittling to him. I shouldn't have said that. That's obviously just what I was feeling at the time. I was probably overwhelmed by the whole situation."

"Nothing good came from Port Arthur," Peter said, which was typically laconic, but punctuated a long reflection upon the day of the massacre. I thought not only of Bryant's murderous vacancy, and the immediate and incalculable agony caused by his slaughter, but also of its broader, fainter and unrecognised contaminations – of husbands who became colder to their wives, and wives who became colder to their husbands. Of shifted relationships between parents and children, now made unbearably tender and fraught, and of all the partners and friends who gradually became alien and burdensome in their private agonies.

We might think of trauma as something that excites communities into tender responses – and it is. But it also strains ordinary intimacies, as the afflicted attempt to resume basic social and domestic duties. There are bills to pay, children to care for, mortgages to service. The best wishes of the community are no guarantee of reintegration, and reintegration is even harder when the origins of the trauma are so violently random.

–

Beaconsfield, Tasmania, is a tiny town, about 40 kilometres north-west of Launceston, where gold was discovered in 1847 and an even larger reef in 1877. A century and a half later, after its gold mine partially collapsed, it experienced the severe and intrusive attentions of the world's media.

At 9.23 p.m. on Anzac Day 2006 – a decade almost to the day after the Port Arthur massacre – a "seismic event" triggered three collapses on level 925 of the mine. "925" referred to the number of metres below ground; in the months before the disaster, blasting and excavations had caused multiple "seismic events" of escalating frequency and magnitude.

Of the seventeen miners then underground, fourteen emerged safely. But three men remained unaccounted for. When the body of Larry Knight was found, a grim assumption was made about the fate of the other two – Todd Russell and Brant Webb. But after three days, contact was made with them: they had survived because of a protective cage, barely large enough to accommodate them, but strong enough to withstand the collapse of 800 tonnes of rock. Russell later told an inquest that he had been about to take a sip of water, when "it's black, it's dark, and we're covered in rock. It happened quicker than what you could blink".

The men were entombed a kilometre below ground, and it was now an unlikely and dramatic rescue story. Hundreds of journalists arrived with their crews. They came from all over the country and from all over the world, and within a prescribed area they unfurled their cables, adjusted their lighting and powdered their faces.

But information, and the sound and vision they needed for their stories, was hard to come by. The mine was selective in what it revealed, which was largely by press release, and the media were contained to an area where sightlines were obscured by plastic sheets. Not that it mattered much – the "action" was occurring a kilometre beneath them.

And so, hoping to fill their stories with weeping faces or emotional testimony, the mob harassed the miners' families and tried vainly to ingratiate themselves with contemptuously reticent locals in the town's pubs. TV producers attempted to bribe workers into smuggling out footage of the mine, while families surrounded themselves with loyal friends who served, with varying degrees of diplomacy, as guards against these insults and intrusions.

In only a few days, the state would mark the tenth anniversary of the Port Arthur massacre, and Peter bitterly reflected on what it took for Tasmania to be paid attention by the mainland's journalists.

—

Peter was part of a small team of paramedics to join the Beaconsfield rescue operation. It was small so that rapport with the trapped miners could be better sustained, and to protect against a catastrophic loss of medics if there was another collapse.

Before entering the mine, Peter was briefed, tested for drugs and alcohol and given his equipment – helmet, harness, resuscitation mask. He brought his own gumboots. The staging area was marked by police tape; outside it, Peter was told, he might be seen by the media scrum.

It took roughly forty-five minutes to descend to level 930 – five metres beneath Russell and Webb. First, there was a lift down to level 375. This part was quick. Then a man with a ute drove him down the spiralling decline to the crib room on level 700, where he placed a location tag to help his own discovery in the event of another collapse, before resuming the slow ride to level 930. Small rocks periodically fell from the roof.

Painstakingly, a small tunnel was bored through to the miners, into which a 90-millimetre tube was fed. Through this tube, a phone line, camera, food, water and medicine were passed to Russell and Webb. On level 930, Peter watched the men on a screen when he wasn't talking to them on the phone.

"One of the first questions they asked me is, 'Is Larry Knight dead?' and I promised myself I wasn't going to bullshit to them," Peter said. "They asked me straight out and I said, 'Yeah, he is,' and they said, 'We thought so, but no one would tell us.' That's just basic – setting up a trust system. They've got to trust us as much as we trust them. You've got to be honest with them, and likewise with all patients. I've never bullshitted a patient, saying 'You're going to be fine' if they're going to die. Probably everyone they've talked to up to that time had avoided saying the word 'Larry', and I think I was just confirming what they'd already guessed."

Peter worked twelve- to sixteen-hour shifts, spending much of the time talking with Russell and Webb. He taught them how to dress their wounds and how to self-inject an anticoagulant to prevent blood clots. He received their urine samples, which were one way of remotely monitoring their health, and suggested stretches they could perform within their tiny and potentially lethal confinement. They talked about music, and after his shift, he carried their messages to the outside world. One message was a half-joking request that *Sunrise* presenter David Koch, of whom Russell was quite fond, did not leave Tasmania until Russell had made it back to ground.

Later, the tube conveyed different essentials: vitamins, Sustagen, handwritten notes from family, and two small iPods loaded with their favourite songs. What *wasn't* fed to them were cigarettes, despite the recurring demands of Webb.

"After a shift, we'd come back to the surface and we went home," Peter said. "There was no debriefing whatsoever, no communication from the ambulance service. When I got home, my wife would be away working her shift at the hospital, and I'd just sleep. Initially I was working every night, but then they made it every second night. So you're one night on, one night off, and throughout the entire rescue no one really knew when these guys were going to come out. You're running tired. I was fatigued to buggery."

We know how the story ends, but of course nobody did at the time. There was no guarantee that the rescue effort wouldn't provoke another fatal collapse, nor was there any firm sense – for the rescuers or the miners – of just how long success might take. This uncertainty – of safety and time – was the crucible they all existed in, and the rescuers had to simultaneously work with great urgency and caution.

The interminability was also something that the miners had to be rescued from, lest they succumb to morbid resignation, and so the paramedics had the dual role of maintaining their patients' morale and physical health. Like the miners burrowing an escape route, the paramedics had to delicately find an equilibrium: sustaining the hope of the men, while remaining honest with them.

"My wife told me that [our young sons] were really good with her," Peter said. "She was really worried, and they both said that I'd be fine. I've always had a bit of a tendency to bullshit to my wife [about the details of his work]. I told her I'd only be working above ground, but she eventually found out that I was in the thick of it. I downplayed things, didn't want her to worry. She's now learnt to read when I'm bullshitting, unfortunately."

After a fortnight of their entombment, the two men were freed. They were "practically crippled", Peter said, their limbs naive and unsteady, but they defiantly left their wheelchairs for their emergence and punched the air.

Peter wasn't on shift then, but he'd been told earlier that if the guys were freed that night, he'd be needed to drive one of them to hospital. The call came at around two in the morning, and Peter collected an ambulance and drove to the site. He was assigned to Todd Russell, who asked David Koch to jump in the back of the ambulance with him. They drove to Launceston General Hospital, where the media had excitedly decamped.

"That morning had the feeling of Christmas morning, or the morning when your first child was born," Peter said. "It was a really good feeling. I went down to my wife's ward after we'd offloaded the guys, just to see her. They'd all been watching it on the news. It was just a moment to share with my wife. Gave her a cuddle, and then she went back to doing what she was doing.

Then the ambulance service took us to the casino and shouted us breakfast."

If the gaze here has been narrowed to Peter's involvement, that's because I've chosen to write it that way, and not because of his self-absorption. Peter becomes awkward and inarticulate when I ask him if he's proud of the rescue. He speaks of all the others who helped and expresses baffled admiration for the skill of those who bored the rescue hole. He said that his father was watching the news on television and wept with pride when he saw his son, but Peter didn't learn of this until after his father's death.

In Peter's home, in the thick portfolios of papers and photos that document a life of service and suffering, the vast bulk of newspaper clippings are about Beaconsfield. It was the story with a relatively happy ending.

—

Friends and colleagues testify to Peter's decline, even transformation, especially over the past five years or so. They describe a once vigorous man who has become reclusive, hypervigilant and morbidly introspective. He is gentle and quiet, but most social circumstances are now intolerable, and small variations of routine can trigger great spasms of anxiety and irritation.

His house is now, emphatically, his retreat. He doesn't often like to leave it, and especially not without his wife, who Peter describes as being like his guardian. "I think she knows me better than I do." When he officially left the ambulance service in 2021, after forty-six years, he wondered what he might do. Someone suggested he work at Bunnings, but Peter couldn't guarantee that he wouldn't explode at an abusive customer.

He considered volunteering at the local cat shelter, but he was filled with an anticipatory sense of grief when he thought about seeing neglected animals. "Grief" was his word. "I don't want to see any more death," he said. "The other day, I moved a moth out of the way of my lawnmower."

"He's disappeared, somewhat," Christine's friend Lisa Bonde said. Lisa is a registered nurse, like Christine, and the two have been close for more than twenty years. She has gotten to know Peter well. "He was here the other day at my house, and a person called in, who he knew quite well," Lisa said. "I was sitting there and just watching, and he sort of shrank into the lounge suite. He disappeared. He doesn't engage, and he gets a look of fear. He is constantly on high alert. If we go out anywhere for lunch, he can't sit facing the door. He's hypervigilant. His whole life has changed.

"For years and years, he was sort of bigger than life. He always had good jokes to tell you. He was always interesting to talk to, because he's right into history and he's travelled a lot. He always had things of interest to talk about. And now, he'll talk to me a lot, but if others are in the room, [or] if he has to move his car out of the driveway, for some reason, and he didn't expect to, he becomes very agitated … He was such a robust man, and so full of life, and now he's sort of like a shell."

Tim Jacobson was Tasmania's state secretary for the Health and Community Services Union and has known Peter for just as long as Lisa – at least two decades. His reflections mirror hers. "Peter was really active with the union," he said. "And I think that he's always been particularly aggressive when it comes to dealing with issues that he felt were unjust. He had rough and tumble relationships with senior management, particularly in Launceston over many years, around certain issues. He's never suffered fools. And he's a highly intelligent man as well. Looking back – because I've known him for a long, long time – I just wonder whether, to some extent, that sort of behaviour could be attributed to even the early signs of his PTSD.

"If you go back through his doctors' reports, his doctors say that he has a number of symptoms: he's a bit intolerant, he's inclined to flare, et cetera. And I just wonder whether, in fact, whilst many people sort of see that as part of his normal behaviour, whether that was some underlying tell in terms of his PTSD going way back.

"He's actually an incredibly gentle man, and when you asked, he was good at opening up and telling you what's going on. But certainly, over the last five or six years, his personality has changed significantly. Particularly since he left the service. He's become more isolated, and more introspective. Seeing this decline, it's been sad. He's not the person he was. And it's hard to imagine he'll ever be that person again."

What has aggravated his injury, Tim said, has been Peter's dislocation of identity, his sense of having been abandoned by Ambulance Tasmania, and the long, brutally adversarial process of claiming worker's compensation.

"Probably the worst aspect in Peter's case, given the high level of need he's had as a patient, is that he's basically had to fight for that care every step of the way," Tim said. "His most recent hospitalisations, he's had to fight on his own behalf to get approval through the workers comp system, even though all the doctors have said that this is what he needs. It's been the insurance company that's been the blocker. [It's] been sinisterly adversarial. These games to avoid costs have been played badly, and I have no doubt that it's added seriously to Peter's injury. And under the surface of all of this, there are still people who treat him like a malingerer."

—

One of Peter's last jobs before retirement made history and national news – and confirmed for him just how damaged he was. It was 11 October 2016, and Peter was in an air ambulance 21,000 feet above the Bass Strait. With him was a woman in labour, only thirty-three weeks pregnant, and her partner.

They had been evacuated from King Island, whose hospital was not adequately resourced to care for such a premature baby. They were trying to fly to Wynyard, on the Tasmanian mainland, but storms obliged them to lengthen their route and land at Launceston.

In the back of an ambulance, the mother might have been offered an analgesic to inhale, but there is no gas on the plane – in the pressurised cabin, there would be a risk of the pilot's intoxication. Then there was the mild G-force of take-off, which

Peter thought had likely encouraged labour, with its downward pressure on the mother's abdomen. Contractions had begun within fifteen minutes of their being airborne, in a plane shaken by turbulence, and Peter understood that he would have to deliver the baby up there among the storm clouds.

On the stretcher bed in the cramped plane, Armando Sonny Day was delivered quickly. He weighed just 2.1 kilograms, and Peter passed him to his father. But something wasn't right. Sonny was blue. Sonny wasn't breathing. "I thought I'd lost him initially," Peter remembered.

Peter chose the smallest mask and resuscitation bag in the plane – both of which were still too large for a premature baby. He held Sonny on his lap, applied the mask and began to ventilate him. It was a delicate procedure – Peter had to be careful not to damage his patient's tiny lungs with overly forceful breaths. He did this for forty minutes – and he wept as he did so. This was unthinkable. "I was totally overwhelmed," Peter said. "I've never been in that position. I did everything that needed to be done, but I paid the price at the end of the case. Crying over a patient that's ventilating – that's the thing that sticks in my memory."

But Peter also remembers the movement of Sonny's tiny tongue – the oxygen was having an effect. They landed in Launceston, and Sonny was saved.

The media were eager to tell the story, and Peter politely consented to interviews and photographs, despite his exhaustion. The reports were framed simply: a feel-good story starring grateful parents and their quick-thinking medic. "If your baby is premature and you are about to give birth on a plane during turbulence 21,000 feet over the sea, Peter James is the man you want at the business end," the ABC wrote.

The stories didn't mention that Sonny had stopped breathing – although some referred to "respiratory difficulties" – or to Peter's crisis of nerve. If you saw Peter on the evening news that night, you would likely have seen a quiet and decent man of few words who was mildly embarrassed by the attention. But knowing Peter, and watching that footage now, he looks blanched. Haunted.

He had delivered, then resuscitated, a premature baby in a cramped plane during turbulence – but Peter could think only of his failure to "bury his emotion". His "resilience had gone out the window", as he put it. He could only think of how he had stood over a baby and wept.

Later, he realised that it was like Broad Arrow again. "In there, you couldn't hear the waves hitting the seawall nearby," he said. "You couldn't hear anyone else talk. There was no noise, no noise at all. You couldn't feel the breeze from the ceiling fans. You didn't feel hot or cold. And time just stopped when you went in there." And so it was on the plane with Sonny. "The thought of losing him was just horrific," Peter said. "I know now how traumatic it was to me because I can't remember hearing any aircraft noise, and normally it's a really noisy environment. It's really weird what your brain cuts out. It's focused on one job – there's no interference from outside."

In that plane, trauma's tattoo pen was at work on Peter's brain. Unlike any previous case, he had imagined – *really* imagined, and therefore felt – the death of baby Sonny. His plates of resilience were slipping, and things were getting through. While Sonny had survived, Peter's imagination had left him with a powerful image – a parallel reality that was intensely experienced and still resonates, ghostlike.

—

In 2017, Peter was referred to Ward 17 of Melbourne's Heidelberg Repatriation Hospital, a psychiatric unit that treats veterans and emergency service workers. It was a six-week admission, and Peter packed his suitcase with a "strange sense of finality, as if I was going to die". He had experienced this sensation before, when packing for a trip to Christchurch, New Zealand, in 2011, to assist in the recovery mission after a major earthquake. "I remember reading somewhere that the troops in the First World War who operated best were the ones that thought they were already dead – who had nothing to lose," Peter said. "I started to feel that."

As Peter sat alone in a waiting room, he cried gently and thought: "So, it's finally come to this." But he accepted his designation as a patient, something he'd witnessed his own patients stubbornly resist. He also had a framework, or a handle to grasp: a diagnosis of PTSD. "Once you have that, you can at least get your head around it and start working on it."

His nurse introduced herself, checked his suitcase and removed the sharp objects. For a man whose toolkit once included scalpels, this might have been an intolerable indignity. It wasn't.

He was now the person requiring help, and he accepted this. They did an MRI scan to rule out degenerative brain disease, thus confirming that his memory loss was likely related to his PTSD.

For six weeks, Peter rose at seven, served himself breakfast from the buffet, then went to mindfulness class at eight. Patients attended tailored classes as well as individual and group therapy. In the evenings, they watched telly together. Another patient's therapy dog often came over and sat on Peter – an Australian shepherd, she had intuited his stress and nightly deposited quantities of her coat onto his lap. "She was bloody gorgeous."

Peter felt comfort in being surrounded by people who understood and shared his suffering. "We treated each other well," he said. "And our journeys might have been different, but the injuries were the same. I do feel bad about the women, though, because it was a pretty blokey environment."

Peter was readmitted to Ward 17 two years later, in 2019, this time for nine weeks and courses of electroconvulsive therapy (ECT). In between, he had received an official medical declaration of incapacity.

Peter wasn't anxious about ECT. He'd seen it administered before as a paramedic, when he'd stand by in case something went wrong, and he was happy to try anything that might improve him. ECT is typically administered as a last resort, after treatment has proved resistant to psychotherapy and medicine, and so it proved with Peter. "I went in, they check your ID number. They put you on oxygen, and you breathe deeply for a little while. Then they give you a drug to put you to sleep, and then there's a muscle relaxant as well, and then they zap you.

You wake up in the recovery room. They don't let you walk back down to the transit lounge. They wheel you. I ended up doing twenty-two lots of ECT, which was a huge amount, and I've got a lot of short-term memory loss from it. That's one of the side effects.

"It didn't go as well as it could have. They put me on to higher doses of mirtazapine [an antidepressant], which gave me a thing called serotonin toxicity. And so while I'm doing the ECT courses, I'm waking up at night and there was a gunman – this is what I was seeing, anyway – coming through the door to shoot me. It was as vivid as anything. I told the veterans on the ward, and they joked they'd just hunt him down and get him. They were good blokes.

"So, I'm having this reaction to the drugs, and these palpitations. My wife used to be a psych nurse, and when I got home ... we've gone straight to the GP and got my meds changed and everything settled down again."

Neither the drugs nor the ECT are cures. But they can soften, mitigate, bevel the edges. They can make intolerable suffering tolerable. Peter said that of everything, the drugs have helped the most. As well as antidepressants, he is on clonidine, a drug usually administered for the treatment of high blood pressure or attention deficit disorder, but which can also usefully treat PTSD-related nightmares. It doesn't seem to stop night terrors, but prevents their being remembered. It has worked for Peter, and he is not woken by them too often these days.

In the evenings, Peter and Christine get comfortable in their lounge room in front of the telly, and Christine will knit and embroider squares that will eventually become quilts. It's a recent and therapeutic pastime, and she looks forward to it after a day working in her hospital's acute physical rehab ward. She has already made a "memory quilt" for her parents on their wedding anniversary, and another to help christen her son's new apartment.

While Christine finds tranquillity embroidering symbols of loved ones' memories, Peter seeks respite from his. But he would also like you to know that there were good times. He helped birth twenty-two children, saved numerous lives, and his profession gave him a great sense of pride and purpose. In the 1970s, he shouted Bob Hawke a beer at Hobart's casino; a few years later, when Hawke was prime minister, Peter saw him again on the tarmac of Hobart's airport. "And he remembered my name," Peter said. "He had a mind like a steel trap. He was a force to be reckoned with, and he was the first Labor PM I voted for in a long time."

Peter pulled a child from the bottom of a pool and breathed life back into her. He delivered a child on an aeroplane. He travelled a kilometre below ground and provided food, water and counsel to trapped miners. He made his parents proud. He made his wife and children proud. He would have made his grandfather proud. And his one long-term goal for his two children was realised: that when they grew up, they'd be mates.

But of all the things he was most proud of in his career, Peter emphasised one – an incident that made sense of his job, justified its attendant mental injuries and confirmed his own value. It was holding the hand of an elderly lady who was dying in the back of his ambulance. "As she was dying, she squeezed my hand. She was frightened. And I was pleased that I was able to hold her hand and give her some feeling of another human being touching her while she passed away. I'll always remember that."

He still doesn't know what else he would have done for a job.

—

Peter was boarding the Manly ferry at Sydney's Circular Quay. It was March 2022, and he was heading back to Sly country, Sydney's Northern Beaches, where he once sat as a boy to watch the breakers and the seagulls.

He was alone, which was unusual. He didn't like to travel anymore, much less without Christine, but this was something he felt was best done on his own. Not that he was really alone, he said, because in the ferry, on his lap, was a backpack that held a steel tin containing his mother's ashes.

Peter's mother Iris died in 2017, two days after he first entered Heidelberg Hospital. Later, Peter and his older sister Dianne agreed to cast their mother's ashes together in the waters of the beaches where they'd spent their childhoods, and where their ancestors had fished and patrolled for endangered souls. A pilgrimage of sorts, and a late homecoming for their mother. But grief, anxiety and a pandemic kept Peter home with his mother's ashes, and then, in 2021, Dianne died of a lung disease. There were times afterwards when Peter stared at an old family photo, all of its members gone now except him, and felt like he was staring at a "void".

Once, his mother had seen his work first-hand. He was driving the two of them to lunch when they saw a head-on crash. Peter rushed to the scene, and his mother was deputised. There was a young man, fatally wounded but not yet dead in the driver's seat. "She was helpful and calm," Peter said. "What I remember is that she had these burgundy boots, and she scratched them and had blood on them. The poor bloke couldn't be saved." They later found out he was a nursing student.

They never spoke about it again. "That might seem weird," Peter said. "I think trauma became my norm. I guess most people would see very little trauma in their lifetime, and it will be a defining moment to them. Paramedics may see it in the morning, get some lunch, then see it in the afternoon."

And now Peter was on the ferry, holding the bag that held his mother and thinking how strange it was that her life had been replaced by a dust that he could carry. He would scatter her ashes tomorrow. He disembarked at the Manly wharf, gripped his bag and began walking to his hotel. He walked up a hill, away from the water, and into the powerful headwinds of memory. The memories were unbearably strong, and Peter began to shake.

"I got into my hotel room and absolutely lost it big time," Peter said. "I sat on my bed and howled. All the memories came back. Bringing my mother back was harder than I thought it would be. After maybe half an hour of sobbing, I called my wife. Then I called my cousin, and he said he'd come and pick me up tomorrow and we'd do it together."

At sixty-three, he was still his mother's son, and his years of exposure to death had not numbed his astonishment about hers. Almost five years had passed, but Peter's journey to these beaches to cast her ashes had made her death freshly disorienting – and he was now insufficiently calloused to fend against the volley of memories that came with it. Trauma had dissolved certain protective membranes. He felt like a hypersensitive antenna, receiving a flood of signals from his boyhood. Beach picnics; fishing for snapper; dawn services on the shore.

That first night in the Manly hotel, Peter took a bottle of wine from his room's fridge, but the medication tasted awful and he put it away.

"The more a man can forget, the greater the number of metamorphoses which his life can undergo," Søren Kierkegaard wrote. "The more he can remember, the more divine his life becomes." But Peter's remembering had become intrusive and cruel, and electrodes and psychotropics could only dull them. He had seen suffering and now suffered in turn, and he felt no divinity. As he lay in bed, his mother's urn on the room's desk, he felt no closer to God. But he'd wondered about Him. Had wondered not so much if God existed, but if he had the capacity for faith – and if he did, whether it might be a comfort, or help him to better understand the chaos that he could never prevent but only bandage.

And as he lay in bed, wishing for sleep, every part of him aching now, he thought of his mother and what she had hoped for herself and for her children, and of the sad, inevitable distance between ambitions and reality. But we do the best we can, he thought, and eventually he fell asleep.

In the morning, his cousin picked him up, and they drove

to Fairlight Beach. Peter waded into the water, holding the urn tightly, focused only on not being imbalanced by the small waves and spilling the ashes. When he was sufficiently far out, the water up to his thighs, Peter emptied the tin.

—

After nine months of long conversations on the phone, I finally flew to Launceston to meet Peter and Christine. He met me at the airport, by the luggage carousel, his eyes large and mournful like a beaten puppy.

After gently shaking my hand, he subtly winced when some children shrieked while playing a game. A quiet man, he radiates an intense fragility, and I realised how generous his collecting me from the airport was: he doesn't leave the house much these days. "It's both my castle and my prison," he told me as we walked out to the carpark.

It was a short drive to his home, where I would spend the night, and on the way we stopped at a lookout. We climbed the narrow, spiralling stairs to the top, where he pointed out the city's landmarks and the places through which he could no longer drive.

Peter and Christine have lived in their house for thirty-one years now. Across the street is the primary school that Sam and Oliver went to, whose flags, when lowered to half-mast after Port Arthur, had once made Peter weep. There was something about the conflation, he told me, of the silent tribute with the children's voices playing in the quadrangle.

It's a large and cosy home, its walls crowded with portraits of distant relatives and old maps of cities. There's a collection of noisy clocks, porcelain plates and military memorabilia: framed-First World War medals and the brass nose of an old howitzer shell. The bookshelves are filled with military histories, and on the wall of the dining room, above a polished mahogany table, is a large portrait of Abraham Lincoln. "A great man of history," Peter said. "'With malice towards none' sums him up."

Peter showed me Christine's sewing room, and next to it the room he has dedicated to his cat Lily, although he concedes that "the whole house is hers". In this sunroom overlooking Mount Barrow, Peter has placed a giant climbing tower for her, and a large box of cat toys, to which he has donated an old pair of his reading glasses she likes to chew. He can speak at length about Lily's vices and virtues.

It was an unusually sunny day, and we walked down the stairs to the large back garden to talk about the book. The week before, I had sent Peter a draft of what I'd written so far, and we would now discuss it, pens and notebooks in hand, sitting on the deck that now covered the old swimming pool he'd anxiously replaced when his children were toddlers. A few feet away was the grave of Daisy, his previous cat.

I was naturally fretful. I'd tried to write Peter's story plainly, but I still wondered if I would have to defend my various digressions, emphases and assumptions. "It's your book, and I trust you," he said simply. I expressed my relief, and then we spent a few hours on the deck drinking tea and going through the manuscript, occasionally correcting numbers or dates, while Peter expanded upon some of his stories.

But reading the draft had unlocked certain memories, including some I'd never heard before. He was still excavating his past, not always voluntarily. "You have got me remembering stuff that I probably had buried," Peter said. "About [my parents'] divorce. One day we were living at Collaroy Plateau, on Sydney's Northern Beaches. My parents had a great argument. I think my mother was having an affair. The next thing I know I'm dragged out to the car with her – she left my sister with my dad. I'm crying that I want to go home. She stopped the car and asked me who I wanted to be with and I said 'Dad'. She returned to the house, dropped me out the front and drove off. She ended up living in Melbourne for a couple of years.

"Me and my sister were terrified that Dad would leave us too. A relative told us that Dad had been found in his car at the Gap, contemplating driving off the cliff. That's when we went to live with Nana. Dad drank a lot after that."

–

The three of us went out for dinner that night, to a place on the harbour. Their shout, they said, and we strode the boardwalk beneath a fullish moon. It was cold now, the tide was out, and the moored boats were lodged in mud.

I felt slightly ashamed that I'd obliged Peter to venture outside so much, although both he and Christine seemed relatively relaxed. In the restaurant, I asked them about their imminent trip to Europe. Their eldest son lived in Prague now, and they would visit him there, then make their way across Europe and, eventually, to Christine's old country of Scotland. Peter was planning a visit to Auschwitz in Poland. I knew of his interest in the Second World War and its cosmic obscenities, but I asked him if he had mentioned this plan to his psychologist.

Peter avoided the implication of my question, and said: "Those that ignore history are doomed to repeat it." I asked more directly: "Does your psychologist think this is a good idea?" He didn't, and nor, it seemed, did Christine. But Peter was determined. After talking about Elie Wiesel's Holocaust memoirs and the diaries of Rudolf Höss, he acknowledged that it might seem like a bad idea, but argued that it wouldn't have the same intense, personally triggering power as Port Arthur.

When we returned from dinner that evening, Peter once again showed me to my room. It used to be Oliver's, and it still had on its walls the posters of his high-school drama productions: *Footloose* and *Little Shop of Horrors*. There was a double bed, a reading chair and a bookshelf stuffed with classics, pulp, travel guides and boardgames. I doubt that it had been touched since Oliver left home.

On the bedside table, Peter had left a glass and a bottle of sparkling water. He hoped there were sufficient pillows and blankets. Throughout my stay, he was sweetly attentive to my comfort. I slept well and woke early the next morning to the sound of rain on the tin roof.

—

Peter and Christine made coffee and toast for me, then took theirs to the lounge room, where they watched *Sunrise* in their slippers and trackpants. I sat beneath Abraham Lincoln at their dining table, where Peter had left a stack of portfolios containing newspaper clippings and other documentary evidence of his career: photos, newsletters, memos, diplomas, citations, clinical notes, memorial cards, printed emails, and the business cards pressed into his hands by reporters at the scenes of various disasters. There was a card, written on behalf of Prime Minister John Howard, inviting him to Parliament House for an event to thank the Beaconsfield rescuers. Peter went and personally thanked Howard for his gun control laws.

There was a document from Ambulance Tasmania, outlining protocols for its members who were joining the international rescue mission in Christchurch. In an appendix, it advised all employees:

> One of the greatest things you can do to help your grieving colleagues is to free yourself from feeling like you have to somehow fix them or take away their pain. You can't do that and people don't want you to try. This means opening yourself to feeling a degree of helplessness – something which makes you a better rather than lesser support! What grieving people frequently want and need is someone with whom they can share their experience at a rate and level that suits them.

There was a high-school report, which bluntly described Peter's achievements in each subject as "ordinary" – except for history, in which he was judged "advanced" – and there were photos of him as a young paramedic, lithe and tanned, looking like Clint Eastwood in an unbuttoned shirt and aviator shades.

I was reading a book of condolence, compiled for Tasmanian emergency workers after Port Arthur, when Peter quietly came into the room. He asked if I wanted anything and expressed his hope that the documents were useful. Then he apologised – as he often did – for speaking too much. Peter was always quick to self-effacement. Before he left, he handed me a short, handwritten note and asked if I thought it would be appropriate if I included it somewhere in the book. The note read:

> To those who could not endure the pain of PTSD any longer: You did make a difference and you do matter. I hope you have found peace.

–

Before Peter dropped me off at the airport, he drove me around a few of the small towns outside Launceston, including Westbury, where Simon Webb lived. Earlier in 2022, not long after our third conversation, Simon had been diagnosed with oesophageal cancer. Peter told me, after I mentioned that Simon's texts had gone quiet – until then, Simon and I had been exchanging book recommendations. Simon's cancer was successfully removed, but the invasive treatment brought a succession of grave respiratory failures. He hadn't left the hospital since and was on a ventilator at Launceston General Hospital when I visited Peter.

I thought it might be nice to see some of the country with Peter, and to visit Simon's town – the place where his itchy soul had finally settled for longer than any other place he'd ever found himself in.

Westbury is an old village that feels forgotten. Thirty years ago, Peter told me, a freeway connecting Launceston with Hobart bypassed it. At 2200 people, it's now smaller than it was 200 years ago, when Irish convicts and refugees from the Great Famine helped found it.

The homes are mostly small shacks. There's a pub, an RSL and a tractor museum. On the main drag, near the hotel, is the impressively grave Catholic church, a large gothic composition of bluestone and slate. It was consecrated in 1874, the same year the colony's statistician recorded: "The average number of Lunatics and Idiots maintained during the year was 353, 200 of whom ... had been Imperial convicts. Of these 353 Lunatics, 270 were kept at New Norfolk, and 83 at Port Arthur."

At the town's southern edge, vast plains spread out from the quiet streets towards the mountains of the Central Highlands. We drove past a large backyard where a few geese were waddling in mud. "Look at them," Peter said, pleased by the image. "I love geese. They won't take any shit from a human."

I saw the small, lush park in which Simon had been walking his dog the last time we spoke. It is across the road from the RSL, which occupies a convict-made building, originally a prison, half a century older than the church. Then we drove down Simon's street. We didn't know it, but at about the same time, Simon's ventilator was being turned off. He was pronounced dead that afternoon. He was seventy-three.

"I've got some good friends here, and it's a nice little town," Simon told me the last time we spoke. "I've got to know a lot of people in a fairly short period of time. This is the place I've lived the longest, actually."

—

A week after Simon's cremation, a small poppy service was held for him at the Westbury RSL club. At the front of the hall, beside the lectern, the club president had arranged a Missing Man Table, traditionally assembled to mark the passing of a veteran. It was a round dining table set for one, and each element had symbolic value. There was a white cloth, empty chair, inverted wine glass. A bread plate with a slice of lemon. Some salt, a poppy and the Bible. There was also a scalloped seashell, the pilgrim's token on the Camino Trail, which Simon had trekked a few years before. And there was Simon's leather pouch, the one slashed by shrapnel in the mortar attack.

An English minister spoke; he had known Simon in the army, where they had energetically discussed faith. He said without malice that Simon was no saint, but he was unusually sensitive to suffering and his life had been a "physical, mental and spiritual rollercoaster". Simon challenged his own faith, Robert said, and debated politics ferociously. "He tried to stir people from their complacency."

An old copper, Rob, a former patient of Simon's who had

become a friend, spoke next. Rob had once reluctantly sought treatment for PTSD. Reluctantly, he said, because he was embarrassed, and it was a long time before he could tell people that he was seeing a psychologist. When he did, he preferred to refer to him as a "cop doctor". Later, he and Simon became friends.

"Simon gently dismantled me," Rob said, "and helped me put the blocks back together. When I told him I was thinking about moving to New Zealand, he said to me, 'So it's your address that's the problem?' That kind of logic annoyed me, but I needed it."

Simon didn't much observe the boundaries that define the modern patient–psychologist relationship – "patients" are known as "clients" today, a word I suspect would have irritated Simon – and in 2018 the two of them cycled the path of the Western Front in Europe. Simon's anxiety was pronounced then, and he was "flustered". "Our relationship changed," Rob said. "And I could help him."

Then there was Nick, a Vietnam veteran who met Simon just two years before at the same RSL club in which he was now eulogising his friend. The poor man seemed to radiate loneliness. "That extreme violence, it creates demons in you," he said. "And you seek answers." Nick wept and seemed lost, perhaps astonished both at the persistence of those demons and at the loss of his sympathetic friend. "We have terrible demons. His are now gone. Captain Webb, you can stand down now. You have gone above and beyond. I will miss his counsel and his friendship."

"Chariots of Fire" played, then the Last Post, and after a minute's silence, mourners were shepherded to the bar where Simon once held court. The building's original structure as a prison remains basically unchanged – inside are six unmodified jail cells.

History is hard to shake. Simon had been repulsed by the war and alienated from its authorities, but this had only brought him closer to it. In complicated ways, the war had determined his life thereafter. He lived with its gravity, sometimes harnessing it, sometimes crushed by it.

"Wasn't Simon's memorial so dignified?" Peter texted me a few days later. "I was impressed. He was a good man."

—

Peter looked out on his back garden recently and watched his clothes hanging from the line. They were all civilian items – t-shirts, shorts, trackpants – and he thought of how proud he was of his old uniform and how conspicuous its absence now seemed. Peter's job had meaningfully defined him, and he liked that definition, but had come to depend upon it. There was a time when his uniform drying on the line had seemed like a private flag declaring his purpose in the world.

But Peter's job now is to forge a new purpose and to recover a sustainable sense of himself, independently of the job that both made and damaged him. And he'll try, while removing moths from the path of his lawnmower.

2

The Copper

BRETT KERSTEN

"I don't know the psychology of it. But everyone was walking around, dead."

They're drinking now, really getting into it – sharing the week's war stories and bitching about command. The coppers called them "nightshift barbies", informal piss-ups for those who'd finished their shifts at 11 p.m., especially on Sundays.

Since his graduation from the Victorian police academy in 1991, Leading Senior Constable Brett Kersten had served in a few stations, each with its own venue for these drinking sessions. In Moorabbin, they used an abandoned courthouse. In the late 1990s in Dandenong, then a hard and heroin-blighted southern suburb of Melbourne, it was typically a footy oval. Just before the shift ended, they'd cruise the area's industrial sites for wooden pallets to use as fuel for their barbecue and gratefully collect donated buckets of KFC and slabs of beer from local vendors. Then the nightshift barbie began.

"We weren't at work, so we could let our hair down," Brett said. "And debrief with a drink. The dark humour was very dark for some of us. We would make out to be funny things that were actually sickening inside."

Police command eventually shut down the barbies. Brett understands why, but he still mourned their passing. "When they stopped that, that's when I noticed the amount of police taking stress leave going through the roof, because they weren't getting the opportunity to debrief," he said. "Getting drunk after a nightshift actually was mentally healthy for them, because they could go over things together – things that had happened over the week ... It depends where you're stationed, and who you're drinking with, but some of my most pleasant memories are drinking with my team. The alcohol had its benefits. It built team camaraderie, but it's a double-edged sword. A lot of the trouble and some of the awful things that happened were as a result of police that had too much drink while in the job."

In the busier stations, Brett said, there was a work hard, play hard culture – a messy cycle of escalating stress and commensurate release. Alcohol might encourage camaraderie, but it can also annihilate – Brett lost police friends in car accidents, their bodies filled with booze.

Then there was alcohol's use on the job as a kind of badge – a sign that one had assumed transgressive powers not prescribed by the Crown. Drinking on shift also had a very specific, practical purpose, Brett said: "Earlier in my career, if you weren't driving around in the divisional van on patrol with an open six-pack between your legs and drinking, if you *weren't* doing that, they'd find a way to get rid of you, because they'd consider you to be an internal investigations department plant. You couldn't be trusted."

At the nightshift barbies, comrades around a fire on a dark suburban oval, sharing slabs and fried chicken, they were bound by the unusual dangers of the job, both moral and physical, and by their gratitude for this moment to exchange stories. But there was one story Brett never shared with his workmates. It's the Dickensian story of his childhood – one of vagrancy, neglect and his eventual admission to a wicked orphanage.

"No, I wouldn't dare share my story with them," Brett said. "I kept my background to myself. Because most of the criminals we're dealing with had the same sorts of backgrounds. You don't want to be tarnished as the enemy."

It was them vs us, crooks vs coppers. His childhood, Brett thought, might confuse these fanatically precise borders – for his colleagues and even for himself. Brett wasn't proud of having overcome his childhood story, or proud of it simply because it was *his* – instead, it was a source of shame, disorientation and a beleaguered self-esteem, one that he has spent a lifetime trying to energetically, and perhaps dangerously, correct.

Privately, Brett also tried to quarantine his past from his own sense of professional competence. But the quarantine was imperfect, and he sometimes wondered if he was dirty, unworthy, stupid – compromised, like the crooks he learned to hate, by the poisons of his childhood.

Later, when the wobbles came, he would ferociously project his own fears onto the "enemy".

—

One of Brett's earliest memories is climbing into his newborn sister's cot and snuggling with her. He'd convince his younger brother Adam to climb in too, and they'd sandwich baby Gabrielle, protecting her from the screams outside their bedroom.

It was 1964, and Brett was almost four. The Kerstens had just moved to Surfers Paradise from Melbourne. Brett is unclear about the reasons for the move, but he assumes his parents had likely "burnt all their bridges in Victoria". Both were violent, unstable – to each other and to their children. His father Anthony was an alcoholic and fitfully employed as a mechanic, brickie, truck driver. He was rarely home, but when he was, he asserted himself with a capricious temper and a belt.

"Reflecting back on that life, [what stands out] was the violence of my dad, the alcoholism," Brett's brother Adam remembers. "My dad didn't like me. He loved Brett. Brett could do no wrong. He kicked my mum down a flight of stairs two weeks before I was born. Trying to get rid of me. Unfortunately for him I was born, and he punished me ever since."

Both brothers said that their parents played favourites, rendering fault lines through the family that still exist today. Brett said that his mother Diane loathed him, and from a young age told him that he'd destroyed her life by obliging her to marry a man she despised when she fell pregnant. She ardently wished he had never been born.

When his parents fought, Brett wedged himself between their legs and pleaded for them to stop. For his interventions, he was often slapped or hurled away. Today, he tearfully accepts that his father was violent, neglectful and chronically resentful, but Brett adored him anyway – his father remained the centre of his world, and Brett deferred to him with dog-like loyalty.

Both parents were bitter captives of their regrets and poisoned by self-pity. Both projected their resentments onto their young children. There was no tenderness in the house, and the children were strangers to physical affection. "Dad had an unfortunate upbringing," Adam said. "There was violence – there were a number of reasons. His dad was very violent, apparently. [My father] had small-man syndrome. He'd start throwing punches as soon as he went into a bar. But he was a very smart man. Maybe too smart to live with his lot. And alcohol ruined things. Had circumstances been different, he could have excelled. Not that I necessarily forgive him for it."

—

One day after school, Brett and Adam returned to an empty house. Their mother and sister were gone. It was 1966. When their father came home a little later, he took them all to the local cop station, where he was told that his wife had returned to Melbourne with Gabrielle.

The boys never went back to school. They soon moved out of their rented apartment, and their lives of vagrancy began. In the mid-1960s, Surfers Paradise was still decades away from the gaudy mass of high-rise hotels that distinguish it today. It was a small and sleepy place, filled with weatherboard beach shacks on stilts. Their father would find a vacant one, break in, switch the power on and deposit his sons there while he vanished on lengthy benders. His disappearances could last days, weeks, sometimes a month.

The boys learnt to fish, making hooks from safety pins and dressing them with discarded bait or with the pippies they found attached to the jetty's underside. Fish were abundant, and the brothers cooked them in their squat and sold their surplus on the street. They searched the bin behind the milk bar and feasted on gooey, partially degraded Violet Crumbles – Brett told me he still retains a preference for slightly rotten sweets.

"We were wild, feral little kids," Adam told me. "I don't know if we ever had a pair of shoes. I remember we burnt out two sets of clippers once when we had a haircut. We were wild kids, and only scared of Dad. We were scavenging for food, breaking into houses. It was a big adventure. But on reflection … I got hepatitis and nearly died. My dad didn't realise.

I turned yellow. Brett took responsibility there. And he realised we needed to be fed. I was five or six. Brett was a little older. He was the big brother, and he took care of his little brother. But at the orphanage later, it was a different thing."

Sometimes the boys would sleep on the beach in tiny caves. At night they'd spy into homes and watch other families eat dinner. They lived like this for years.

"On occasion, Dad would come back, but when he came back it was always very late at night," Brett said. "I'd always wait up. I wouldn't sleep enough, because I was waiting, hoping my dad would come back. My brother at that stage was only four or five, so he would sleep. And if my dad did come back, he'd always come back with two longneck bottles of beer, one for me, one for him, and we'd sit on the steep step overlooking the beach, and we'd have a bottle of beer each. On reflection, he was always drunk – pretty blind drunk, actually."

Then, in 1969, their mother reappeared. They hadn't seen her since she'd left, and at first Brett didn't recognise her. She announced that she was taking the boys back to Melbourne. And she did – but she would soon abandon them again, which was when Brett and Adam were fatefully entered into the Christian Brothers' orphanage in South Melbourne. It would prove much worse than their life of vagrancy.

–

The boys played marbles in the courtyard while the vampires watched. That's what the Christian Brothers looked like to Brett, with their forbidding auras and black, ankle-length cassocks. They seemed to malevolently glide through the orphanage, never touching the ground.

Of course, you'd never call them a vampire to their face – their authority was fanatically guarded and brutally expressed. They were guardians of lost boys and tenders of the Lord's flame, but plenty of the Christian Brothers were also bullies and child rapists or protectors of child rapists.

Brett and Adam, unwanted by their mother and father and then rejected by their grandparents, now found themselves in the St Vincent de Paul Boys' Orphanage in South Melbourne. There were about 120 boys then, few of them technically orphans – most were abandoned or severely neglected children. They lived with few possessions, slept in large dormitories and showered communally under the aberrant gaze of the vampires. In the local pubs and milk bars, collection tins for the home were filled with the public's spare coins.

Already, by the late 1960s and early '70s, this style of institution was anachronistic. Out-of-home care was being replaced by foster care. But the Catholic Church stubbornly resisted this change, more so than other denominations, persisting with its large orphanages until late into the decade. It did not want to relinquish either its significant financial investments in the homes or its captive audience for indoctrination.

And so, to the home on Cecil Street Brett and Adam went. The place resembled a prison, with its high walls laced with barbed wire and shimmering with the shards of broken glass that were mixed with its mortar. The resemblance extended to the home's tribal systems of patronage and protection, and immediately the brothers began figuring out their place in the violent hierarchy of their peers. This was much easier for Brett than for Adam, given he was an unusually large and strong boy while his younger brother was conspicuously small and frail. Physical size and ferocity were assets in the dorms, not only against the other boys but against the predatory Brothers.

Brett's home number was 48. Adam's was 89. These numbers were sewn into their uniforms and, said Adam, "tattooed in my head". The boys were up at 7 a.m., for two-minute showers with no shampoo. Breakfast was cereal, porridge and toast served with a pot of tea. There were six boys to a table, and always too few satchels of Vegemite between them.

They swept their dorms and polished the Brothers' shoes. Each Sunday they sat in the pews and crossed themselves and quietly heard the recitals of rites:

"Brethren, let us acknowledge our sins, and so prepare ourselves to celebrate the sacred mysteries ... I confess to almighty God and to you, my brothers and sisters, that I have greatly sinned, in my thoughts and in my words, in what I have done and in what I have failed to do, through my fault, through my fault, through my most grievous fault; therefore, I ask blessed Mary ever-Virgin, all the Angels and Saints, and you, my brothers and sisters, to pray for me to the Lord our God."

As the senior altar boy, Brett helped prepare the chapel for mass. As he did, he filled his pockets with the communion bread so that he wouldn't go hungry later.

—

The orphanage was materially austere, and there were few books or toys. Any toys that might be sent to an individual boy and held in his private possession would be violently desired by others, and often more trouble than it was worth.

Bed-wetting was considered a punishable offence by some of the larger and more sadistic boys – something sick and weak and deserving of a bashing. Nor did you want to be thought a "poof". Like the bed-wetters, anyone labelled such was subject to severe beatings. "The trick," Brett said, "was staying out of the spotlight."

Brett planned his escape, which included hitchhiking back to Queensland to find his dad. "My whole world and my loyalty was to my father," he said. "In my mind, I worked out that Queensland was probably 1000 miles north. I had a good idea which way was north. We were locked in at night, there were big fences around the orphanage, but I didn't think I'd have any problem getting out. So, my plan was to escape."

On the beaches of Surfers Paradise, he'd developed confidence in his wiles, and he possessed a child's expansively hopeful imagination. What prevented him from attempting escape, he said, was the impossibility of taking his brother. Refusing to abandon Adam, Brett shelved his plans and instead, most nights after the lights went out, banged his head on the wall above his bed. Sometimes, late at night, Brett and Adam could hear the Brothers creep into their dorm room and into the beds of other boys.

Brett became an accomplished fighter. Few boys would challenge him. Alone, anyway. But sometimes, groups would attack him. One "vivid memory", he said tearfully, is of being overwhelmed by a group of five boys and seeing his tiny younger brother running towards the scrum, trying to push the aggressors off him. "I was so proud," he said. "I was his protector, but now he was protecting me."

"Me being a strong boy and a fighter," he said, "you would have boys under your protection. So if there were some bullies that would attack my brother or boys in my protection, they know that I'd be coming for them ... You never touched a young brother of a bigger boy, and so [Adam] was protected. That didn't mean I didn't get in fights, but there was a pecking order, and the fight would always be with me or boys of my stature ... I'd have to be the strong one to keep that sort of status quo."

Adam said that Brett protected him well during their years of vagrancy. But his recollection of their time in the orphanage diverges painfully – and irreconcilably – from Brett's. "He was a gang leader," Adam said. "And he could make boys do horrible things to me. He looked after me outside. But in the home it was different."

–

The boys didn't often see their parents – they rarely visited. Nor did they ever see their young sister, Gabrielle. Occasionally, letters arrived, most often from their father and addressed to Brett, but the Christian Brothers vetted correspondence, and most of the letters were withheld – decades passed before Brett received them. He declines my request to see the letters. He says they're too ugly.

Whether as gang leader or noble protector, Brett was fierce enough to ward off the predations that some Brothers practised brazenly on other boys. "Brother Rex Elmer, I saw him molest boys," Brett said. "The worst Brother was John Francis Coswello. He raped boys in the showers."

Many years later, Brother Elmer would be convicted, on three separate occasions, of sexually abusing children in his care, including a boy whose father had murdered his mother. Elmer's most recent conviction was in 2021, when he was seventy-six, an insomniac with a weak heart and resected bowel. When sentencing him, the judge weighed his frailty against the aggravating qualities of his crimes, not least his considerable authority and the vulnerability of those submitted to it. "You took advantage of and contributed to the wretched life that each of these boys endured as orphans," Judge Claire Quin said. "Some twenty years ago, Judge Neesham in this Court said of your offending against twelve boys in the same position: 'It requires little imagination to put oneself in the place of any one of your victims. Here was an adult, a man in authority, a man of God, doing what they no doubt believed to be their private acts that were intrusive, obnoxious, frightening and wrong. They believed they were helpless. Who could they tell? Who would believe them? It is little wonder that all your victims bear deep emotional scars to this day as is vividly borne out in their statements.'"

Adam said that, as a boy, the abusive horrors of the place were absorbed and normalised. It was simply the state of the world, grim and unfortunate, perhaps, but he had nothing else to compare it to. He couldn't grasp the aberrance or sickness of what he'd experienced, because there was no point of contrast. And so he measured himself poorly, concluding that he deserved the cruelties, or, at least, was an inferior boy for so passively accepting them.

But then, one day, Adam glimpsed a sign that all of this was deviant. "There was one day in Form 2 or 3, and a Christian Brother was teaching us – Brother Shirley, who reminded me of the singer Rick Springfield. And I thought: why did he become a Christian Brother? He was a violent young bloke. He used to punish kids. You'd kneel down on the dais, and he'd use a blackboard compass with wingnut bolts and belt you on the arse. It nearly put you through the blackboard. Anyway, one day, someone knocked on the door – and he shoved the compass up his habit. Well, that was the penny dropping for me. Why is he hiding the compass? They all do it. And it's dawned on me that *he's not allowed to be doing it*. It's not normal. That's when I rebelled more, at least in my head. This is all wrong. Do people outside know this is happening? By the time I left the place, I'd come to understand: it was all wrong from the start."

–

The brothers experienced a hard and peculiar education. Their development, in some ways, was accelerated by their abandonment. Precociously, they learnt to survive. They don't speak to each other much these days, but they both use the word "adventure" to describe these early years. But this was hardly compensation for the loss of parental love, even if neither brother looks upon that time as traumatic.

Their admission to the orphanage was another great disruption, and the "adventures" of vagrancy were replaced by severe institutional control. These were very different experiences, but they shared a theme: the violent indifference of adults who were meant to care for them.

In the orphanage, the boys learnt little beyond their primal conditioning. They developed a hypersensitivity to threat and learnt, in response, how to either fight or camouflage themselves. They may also have deepened a bitter sense that no one cared about them, and that it was therefore always best to look out for yourself – if that "self" wasn't already too worn and precariously defined to be worth protecting. After all, before the Kersten boys reached puberty, their own parents, grandparents and the Church had all brutally forsaken them.

In a more formal and practical sense, the boys received a terrible education. They learnt nothing about sex, romance, finance, nutrition, driving, employment, politics ... this list could go on indefinitely. "We were so removed from reality and how the real world worked," Brett said. The Christian Brothers, as custodians of these lost boys, did not see their job as preparing them for the world beyond those high walls. It was their job to secure the boys' faith in their Lord and Saviour, and beyond that – well, good luck to you.

When Brett turned fifteen, he was called to the principal's office. He was surprised to see his mother there, and then was shocked to learn that he was being kicked out – fifteen was the age of automatic eviction. Out by the weekend, they told him. It was Friday.

"Have you thought of a job?" the principal asked.

Brett stared dumbly. A job? How was he supposed to get a job? Did he really have to leave immediately?

"And do you have somewhere to stay?" the principal continued.

To this, at least, Brett had an answer: over the years, his mother had promised that upon release, he could stay with her. But now that Brett mentioned it, his mother became hysterical: there was absolutely no room for him with her.

"I was devastated," Brett said. "It pulled the rug from under my feet."

Brett was given a newspaper and told to look for jobs in its classifieds. He was soon offered a job as a storeman in a shop that sold car parts.

He was also given the address of an elderly lady who'd offered her name as a potential host of released boys needing a roof and steady meals. Brett appeared on her doorstep one day, carrying everything he had – about 60 cents in his pocket and a suitcase holding some spare clothes. The woman seemed shocked and irritated and told him she had only nominated herself because others at her church had done the same. She had never expected, nor desired, the actual appearance of a boy. Brett impressed upon her his desperation, and she begrudgingly yielded, but her hostility made his boarding untenable. One Sunday, when Brett refused to attend mass with her, she denounced him as a child of Satan.

So, Brett left. He had a job but no house and partially reverted to his earlier life of vagrancy. That winter, he slept on a bench in the Brighton cemetery. He felt safe there, he said, with its old trees and grandly fenced perimeter. And at night, it was quiet. He worked during the days and saved enough to buy a bicycle. In the morning, he'd ride the few kilometres from the graveyard to the car parts shop.

The world was baffling to Brett, and he missed his brother. He was also badly malnourished. But he was saving, at least. First, there was the acquisition of the bike. Then a 1962 Holden, purchased for $99, which he learnt to drive with the help of his boss. It also replaced the cemetery as the place where he now slept.

"[My] boss was a good man," Brett would later write. "He wanted to look after me. His wife had died and he asked me to come and live with him. I distrusted men as a result of my experiences in the orphanage. I didn't trust men in fear of being raped. This made it impossible for me to have close mates and male friends. I believe that I missed many opportunities for good friendships and also life opportunities because of this fear."

He found a place to rent in Fitzroy Street, St Kilda, and then another job, better paying, as the driver of a removal truck. But he was getting weaker. The ingenuity, the self-sufficiency he'd developed as a boy in Surfers, had deserted him. He lost significant weight. Then he lost his job. "It's a devastating thing to be sacked," he said. "It's a great discredit to you."

For a week, he lay in bed, convinced he was dying but serenely resigned to the fact. He experienced euphoria, flickered in and out of consciousness. This parlous state, he said, was the result of his institutionalisation – he had not developed the ability to feed himself properly, nor the trust to ask others for help.

He was rescued by a fellow orphan boy who had been released a year after he was. He came and made Brett strong coffee with lots of sugar, then, over days, fed him baby food. Brett survived. Grew stronger. He found another job – this time as a storeman in the bookshop of the Caulfield Institute of Technology.

By now, Adam had turned fifteen and been evicted from the home. He came and lived with Brett. Brett saw himself as a father figure and tried to act like one, drawing on what he remembered seeing on *The Brady Bunch*. It was a "steep learning curve", he said.

While the brothers are not close these days, each accepts the other's account of how the orphanage helped forge their different personalities. "At the start, Brett was more anti-authority in the boys' home," Adam said. "He was very tough. Could take on five kids at a time. He didn't appear to be scared of the kids, or the Christian Brothers. But Brett became more institutionalised than I did."

Brett accepts this. He agrees that he came to internalise the strict regimens of the orphanage and would later seek the institutional shelters of the military and police force. He would place great faith in the state, in the royal family, in the law and authority generally. It was very different for Adam, who nurses a powerful contempt for and suspicion of governments – for most forms of authority, in fact. He has refused to engage the public redress scheme for institutional abuse victims, for example, just as he "refused to get vaxxed". "I saw another agenda," he said. "I live in my bubble these days. A lot of us kids have taken it all through our lives. We were broken from the start."

Knowing this, it was five years before Brett told his brother that he was a cop. Adam became a boilermaker. He also worked on farms, and in abattoirs, installing their machines. He is a man obsessed by and gifted in engineering. Today, he restores vintage cars for collectors, and told me that there are few days when he's not in overalls. Like his brother, Adam found his purpose in work.

—

The St Vincent de Paul Boys' Home finally closed its doors in 1997, when the Mary MacKillop Foundation assumed occupancy. The foundation is still there today, helping the old boys access their files or counselling. It was decades before either brother physically returned.

Brett went first. He was, by then, a copper, and while out on patrol he happened to drive past. He decided to go in and introduce himself. Brett was told he could apply to see whatever papers they had on file for him – school records, photos – which he did. Adam, learning of this, tentatively decided to return too. "Probably into my forties, I didn't much think about those days," Adam said. "I had a career, mortgage. But when you finally pay off the house, or almost pay it off, life becomes a little more comfortable – you find you have free time, and the mind has free time, and those things pushed aside once pop up. Probably in my mid-forties I struggled with my past. I had a lot of anger. A lot of disappointment in the government."

Adam was anxious about returning, he said, although the MacKillop staff were gentle with him. Still, things went badly. "I had an adverse reaction," he said. "It surprised me. I thought I was tougher than that. That I had thick skin. To deal with the Christian Brothers – it'll make or break you. I thought it had toughened me. But I had a bad reaction. Though I kept going back for two years to talk with Katrina [a heritage officer] – and she was an angel. But eventually I stopped. It was the same thing, over and over: I was just screaming at this woman. That poor lady put up with a lot from me. But it was a good experience in a way, because I didn't have photos, school reports, those things – I had no signs of my childhood."

The photos he received from MacKillop's heritage officer were revelatory for Adam. They helped vanquish his long-held guilt, his lingering sense that he was a shameful coward. Upon seeing those photos, the reality of his situation in the home became starkly obvious – and suddenly the fog of his emotional memories, the way his guilt had retrospectively altered his sense of the experience, lifted. Adam had carried with him, well into middle age, a sense that his abuse was somehow the product of his own weakness, the natural consequence of his pathetic incapacity to protect himself. Seeing the photographs changed that.

"I saw a photo of me as an eight-year-old, and things really hit home," Adam said. "I'm a little bloke. One of the smallest in the place. But I had blamed myself because I saw kids fight back and I didn't. *What a pathetic thing you were to not fight back*. But seeing that photo, it all came crashing home. I'd been beating up on myself for so long – but how can a tiny little kid fight back? I also realised: it wasn't personal. It was an attack against kids. The Christian Brothers saw their job [as breaking] our spirit. Not mine, but *all* the kids."

It is a common quality of childhood abuse: the young victim, in their innocence, internalises the moral squalor visited upon them. A self-punishing assumption is made, either consciously or subconsciously: something awful happened to me, and therefore *I* am awful. For the child, the distinction between perpetrator and victim can collapse entirely. In the victim's mind, there is only a sense of repugnance and a stench of transgression, and a belief that they must, somehow, have encouraged the abuse. This sense of complicity can be powerfully imagined and accepted as real deep into adulthood; the shame becomes a lingering trace element of the original abuse.

—

Unsurprisingly, Brett's self-esteem was also poisoned. His experience of the world had insistently suggested that he was unworthy of love, guidance or support. His capacity for trust had also been corrupted, and this made relationships, including a romantic or social life, very difficult. He possessed a medley of assumptions that repelled intimacy: *I'm not worthy of love; I don't understand love; and even if I was worthy and understood, they will leave anyway, because everyone leaves.*

"It took years, took me probably into my thirties, before I let people close to me," Brett said. "Because in the orphanage, and with my father, anyone you got to know would move on. In the orphanage, kids would be adopted out, or their families would come back and get them. There'd never be a goodbye, they're just gone. So, you tended to sabotage your relationships. If anyone got too close, you'd stop it. And that was your way of being in control and not getting hurt. It took me a long time to get through that and over that and realise that people would naturally get close to me, and I'd always sabotage it. And I'd think: why haven't I got long-term friends? I realised I had a problem. I need to change something I'm doing.

"My first wife, I never stopped loving her. But I couldn't cope with her loving me so much. And in hindsight, it was probably because I was scared of losing her that I pushed her away. If that makes sense? It took a lot of years to start to put things together – [realising] that your life has been ruled by fear, subconsciously, [and that] there's so many things you're traumatised with that it's hard to trust anyone."

—

In 1985, Brett joined the army. Upon his recruitment, he felt a wash of confidence – a sense that he was fit to join something important. This sense of his own capacity, and the army's reflected faith in it, was enormously pleasurable.

Then, under a profane sergeant, he was subject to a breaking down, a hazing, a dismantling before reconstruction. And he loved it. "I saw why they were doing it," he said. "It wasn't until I joined the army that things changed. I started to see the bigger picture, and I started to take pride in myself. They tend to break you down in the army. Well, they did in those days. You go to the recruiting office, and you do the exams and the tests, and if you get in, they tell you that you're the cream of the Australian population, you're the best of the best. And so you get that sort of elevated sense – it puffs the confidence up a bit. And then you get to the army, and you're met at the gate, usually by an overbearing sergeant. He'll be spitting in your face as he's screaming. 'You oxygen thief! You're ten steps lower than a snake's belly!' And they break you down mentally. But as they train you, they build up your confidence that, well, you're one of the best soldiers in the world now."

Brett could feel the strange, empty places inside him filling with something substantial. Initially, sure, there were peaks and valleys – flattered by the army's acceptance, he then submitted to the corporal's withering tongue. But whereas the orphanage's cruelty had felt senseless, in the army he could glimpse the brutality's purpose. It was making him a soldier, and he was making a self – earning a sense of community and competence. Army life gave Brett a strict and predictable routine, which he cherished, and it suited his capacity for devotion and hard work. It also allowed him to dream of himself as a "contributor" – a participant in something much larger than himself. Something with a history. Something that was respected. And something that stressed the sanctity of control.

Brett said he did well in the army – was told he had leadership qualities; was groomed to be an officer. But he had also fallen in love and become engaged, and he thought the military life would not support a married one, especially when he was on a 24-hour standby for deployment. After almost four years, he left the army and returned to driving trucks.

The engagement didn't last, and neither did Brett's satisfaction with civilian life. The uniform beckoned, and he applied for the police academy; he was accepted and found himself the oldest there among the prospective cadets.

—

It was 1999, about midnight, and their shift had just begun. Brett and his partner were patrolling Dandenong, in Melbourne's south-east. Things were quiet. Few people were out. They cruised around the train station's carpark. Nothing was happening. The radio was silent. Across the road from the station, there was a cluster of shops – chippies, barbers, suburban accountants – all of them shut. Brett drove down the narrow laneway that ran behind them. Everything was dark and still.

Brett is agnostic about premonitions, but he uses the word to explain his impulse to stop the patrol car halfway down the laneway. He'd seen nothing, heard nothing. Neither had his partner. The decision to stop was just ... *a feeling*.

"Stay here," he told his partner. "I'm gonna take a look behind these shops."

And there she was. He still refers to her as the Christmas tree angel, and he found her in the yellow light of his torch behind a shop. She was unconscious, lying face down in vomit. Brett checked her pulse and breathing – both were dangerously faint. He moved her into a recovery position, and she gasped. "I observed she wasn't the usual-looking heroin addict I was used to seeing," Brett said. "This girl looked about fifteen years old. She was small in stature. Maybe less than five feet tall. She was tiny. She was unusually pretty. The heroin hadn't taken its toll on her like I had seen with other heroin addicts. She wasn't scabby, dirty, hollowed-out the way heroin addicts often end up. I imagined she could have doubled as a Christmas tree angel. The type of decoration you would put at the top of your Christmas tree."

The angel gasped, told Brett to fuck off, then fell unconscious again. He called for an ambulance.

—

By now, Brett had been on the job several years. He was hardened, often numb; compassion had largely been conditioned out of him, both by the prevailing cultural suspicion of it as an operational and personal weakness, and by daily exposure to hardened criminality and its consequences.

In those days, Brett said, Dandenong was run by drug dealers. Heroin was cheap and ubiquitous. Few shifts went by without an overdose, a drug-related assault or both. Pricked by needles, spat upon and bitten by addicts, Brett submitted to countless blood tests during his career. He saw the elderly bashed and robbed for drug money; he saw the domestic squalor and neglect of children in addicts' homes. He came to see addicts with an uncompromising brutality, as people whose submission to the needle had evaporated all charm, grace and any ambitions unrelated to scoring the next hit. As Brett saw it, addiction winnowed its subjects to a mere appetite – and in trying to satisfy it, debased not merely themselves, but society.

He hated them. They were zombies, he thought, a word he used a lot. "I had learnt to hate drug addicts," he said. "So many families and lives were destroyed by them. I had made up my mind years earlier that any idiot stupid enough to stick a syringe in themselves and inject themselves with illicit drugs doesn't deserve to be treated as human. To me, they stopped being human the moment they took that first hit of heroin. They don't deserve the compassion and care I would normally give to anybody else. They were just zombies to me."

Most days, Brett saw something that ratified this belief and consolidated his increasingly consumptive hatred. But now, next to the Christmas tree angel, his compassion was stirred again. He was determined to save her.

–

The girl's breathing was alarmingly shallow and laboured. Before the arrival of paramedics, she flickered several times between consciousness and unconsciousness. When she roused, she swore at Brett. Called him a cunt. He kept his hand on her back, assuring her that help was on its way. In her addled state, she didn't realise how urgently she required it.

The wait for the paramedics felt interminable to Brett. He didn't think it consciously at the time, but as he waited, he was deeply absorbing the dissonance between the squalor around him and the physical suggestion of innocence he saw in the young woman. It was an image that would haunt Brett, containing, as it did, two things he'd once thought incompatible.

The ambulance arrived. Brett said he always got on well with paramedics – they were comrades who paid the same psychic taxes as coppers. But on this job, things got tense. The Christmas tree angel, roused again from unconsciousness, spat in the face of one medic. She was violently refusing their attentions, their stretcher, their lift to the nearest hospital – and that evening, the medics did not have the patience to persuade or coerce her.

"If she doesn't want to get in the ambulance, she can stay here," they told Brett.

"I shouldn't have been surprised," Brett said. "The local ambos were just as burnt out as we were. We were both attending overdoses every day. They too had had enough of the druggies … But I had decided that this girl was going to live … If they left without her, she would die."

And so Brett insisted. The angel was placed upon a stretcher and loaded into the back of the ambulance. Once there, she found the strength to kick one of the medics in the face.

—

Brett's shift finished at 7 a.m. His next began at 3 p.m. His first job that afternoon was to attend a stabbing at Dandenong Hospital, which was where the Christmas tree angel had been taken that morning. While there, Brett inquired about her condition.

He was told that she had technically died seven times that morning but was revived each time, and around 7.30 a.m. had ripped the tubes and monitoring devices from her body and walked out.

"I felt pleased with myself," Brett said. "I had found her accidentally and kept her alive and breathing until the ambulance and help arrived."

A fortnight later, Brett was at the police station's kitchen table, drinking a cup of tea. That's how he started most shifts – nursing a cuppa while savouring the tranquillity of those few minutes before it all began again. He could see through to the station's holding cells, where detectives were speaking solemnly with a young woman: the angel.

Brett gestured for one of the detectives – an old friend – to come over so that he might discreetly ask what was happening. The detective told him that the angel had just been arrested for violently robbing an old woman at the local train station. The angel, he said, had forced the woman to hand over her purse by threatening her with a blood-filled syringe; then, having received the purse, jabbed the woman anyway and pushed her off the platform. The woman was in her eighties and broke her hip.

"I felt angry," Brett remembers. "Angry with myself. I am still angry with myself. I had let my guard down. I had let compassion and my sense of duty enable this [attack] to happen. The guilt that I've worn all these years because I showed compassion, because I saved that young girl's life, and that's what she went on to do. If you wonder why police are so hard and don't show compassion, it's because it's come back to bite them ... People are often critical of police for lack of feeling and compassion. People are critical of why we become desensitised. But is it any wonder we become so numb? Too often we let our guard down. She was anything but an angel. She was just another zombie, preying on the innocent and vulnerable. Sometimes, in anger and frustration, I wish that other people could have a try at walking in a policeman's shoes. I am sure they, too, will become numb to feelings of compassion for those zombies."

Brett leaves the implication of his reaction unspoken, but it's as obvious as it is heavy: that he should have left the angel to die. That he considered this not only possible but desirable is disturbing; his sense that he had a god-like influence over her fate was revealed when he said, "I had decided that this girl was going to live."

In this world, Brett said, you develop hardened instincts, and see any deviation from them as a weakness. You develop a combatively unnuanced morality, and you act upon it. The world is brutal, and brutally schematised: "It was us versus them," Brett said. "We had no sympathy for crooks. It was severe. We were programmed to think there's three kinds of people: there's police, victims and the enemy. And you had no quarter for the enemy."

Most people might comfortably accept that in saving a stranger's life, the rescuer does not assume responsibility for what that stranger does next. The rescuer has fulfilled a grave duty without prejudice, no more or less. They cannot be condemned for not seeing the future. Most of us do not fretfully consider our role in outcomes we could not possibly have foreseen. Perhaps this is because for most of us, the decisions we make at work don't have such potentially severe consequences.

But Brett absorbed a different lesson. When he talks about the angel and her rescue, he talks about "compassion" and "professionalism" as two different, even incompatible, things – compassion is a weakness that can have terrible consequences. Were he to frame the rescue of the angel as humane professionalism, the torturous psychic loop in which he found himself might have been avoided. Instead, in imagining that he could and should have prevented the old lady's trauma, he assumed creepily god-like powers over life and death. Brett had been taught, by culture and experience, to suspect his own compassion – and the assault of this old lady had painfully reinforced that lesson.

—

There's a sour irony that those who enter certain vocations with a pronounced sense of public duty, and a desire to protect or to alleviate suffering, can, through repeated exposure to human depravity, become numbly detached from their initial motivation. Here, again, is moral hazard: by professionally practising your beliefs, you can become estranged from them – and from yourself.

In all of my conversations with Brett, the word "compassion" recurs. Its recurrence is significant, in part, I think, because Brett has never settled upon its worth or upon his capacity for it. He suffers from an awkward ambivalence, an unreconciled tension between his feeling that compassion is necessary and virtuous, and his feeling that it is also adjacent to weakness and naivety. For Brett, compassion is a curiously charged and dangerously bipolar impulse, simultaneously holding the potential for love and injury.

Brett has suffered, in different moments, from feeling too much and feeling too little. He can speak proudly about both a surfeit and an absence of compassion. He could be disturbed by an abundance of sorrow, as when he held a dying person in his arms; yet in other moments he could be struck by his cool absence of feeling and he would wonder who he might be.

In his first year as a cop, he received a call in the divvy van: a local restaurant's alarm had been triggered. Brett and his partner heard the alert just as they were passing the address. It was early morning, not long before dawn. The restaurant's front door had been busted open, and they cautiously entered. Immediately, they smelt petrol. Then, Brett saw a man in overalls and a ski mask emptying a jerrycan.

"He appeared to look up at us and panic," Brett said. "I could smell the strong odour of petrol covering the whole length of the floor space as he lit the match. Immediately, he and the restaurant went up in flames. The whole place completely engulfed. I watched him for possibly a few seconds before I was driven back by the heat.

"I don't think the arsonist intended to burn himself to death. I think he panicked and just didn't think before he lit the match. He was definitely at the wrong end of the restaurant. There was no way he could escape.

"We weren't compassionate police in those days. We were conditioned not to be. I had no feeling for this arsonist. He didn't scream for long. One less arsonist meant one less oxygen thief to me. Now, all these years later, I feel a sense of guilt. I still have no feeling for that arsonist. There was nothing I could do to save him. But I feel guilt that I had no feeling for him at all. Was I that broken myself?"

—

Brett has sought jobs and institutions that valorise control – that are, in fact, defined by it. Like Peter James, his identity, for a long time, was bound intimately to the belief that he might benignly control unstable situations. Specifically, he needed to believe that he was capable of maintaining self-control. His self-conception hinged upon proving to himself that he was sufficiently smart, brave and competent to honour his uniform and transcend any personal doubts, and thus maintain peace and stability.

But things happen. Obscene things that are beyond your control. One night, while stopped at a red light, Brett and his partner saw a Commodore zoom through the intersection at great and illicit speed. When their light turned green, they followed.

"We travelled perhaps half a kilometre along the road when I first noticed the tree up ahead," Brett said. "There seemed to be car debris scattered around it. As we drove closer, I could see a lot of debris. Then I saw the other tree and the red Commodore wrapped around the base of it. There were people in the Commodore, but there was no movement. We immediately called on the radio for an ambulance and fire units. Our local divisional van came up in reply: they were also on their way."

Brett and his partner parked and got out of the car. There was no noise – it was eerily still. As they got closer, Brett intuited the reason for the silence, and his body failed him. "As I approached and looked into the car, my feet stopped working perhaps five feet away," he said. "I couldn't move. It was as if my feet were bolted to the spot. The top half of my body was trying to lurch forward and to rush in and help. I did not understand what was wrong with me. Then, as if in sudden realisation, I knew what was wrong with me. What I was seeing in the car wasn't making sense in my head. What I was seeing was perhaps five, maybe six bodies. They were so intertwined and mangled, I could not see where one body finished and the other one started."

The carnage was so violently surreal that it was disorienting – as if Brett had stepped into a parallel universe where the laws of biology and physics were grotesquely changed. "Fight" and "flight" are long accepted stress responses; a third, more recently researched, is "freeze". Here, Brett was experiencing the latter. "This is just one example of when I experienced brain and body dysfunction," he said. "Where I wanted to rush in and help, but my feet would not let me. My brain could not make sense of what I was seeing. I am still haunted by many incidents and visions I witnessed over my career. I think what saddens me and weighs heaviest is my sense of helplessness on these occasions. Police are trained and programmed to take control and be in charge. This incident, like many others, I could not control."

–

When Brett was twenty-two and recently married, he drove with his wife Lucy to Queensland in search of his father. Despite everything, Brett was still tethered to him – less powerfully, perhaps, than when he was younger, but some love and loyalty had survived.

They went to his father's old drinking haunts, asked around about his whereabouts. And they found him. He was living in a caravan and still hopelessly lashed to the bottle. Brett found that his father had debts all over town; Brett squared a few of them. He bought him groceries. But his father was still bitter, vindictive – especially after a drink. One evening, he asked to see his son's hands. After Brett held them out, his father sneered: "You've never worked a day in your life. You've got girl hands. You're still just a little Jewish boy, your mother's son."

They nearly belted each other, and that was that: Brett and Lucy left. Brett would never see his father again. Letters were exchanged – usually caustic ones from his father – and while

Brett always vaguely hoped that proper contact would be re-established, it never happened. In 1993, two years into his police career, Brett received a call telling him that his father was dead.

Brett drove, once again, to Queensland. He organised a funeral service there, and then another in Melbourne. He spoke at both funerals and said that he was happy to eulogise his father without bitterness. "I prefer to only speak of the good and positive of people," he wrote to me. "Anything negative I would prefer not to speak. I am widely known for, and possibly respected for, not talking negative of people. Especially the dead."

I asked Brett if he remembered how he'd eulogised his father, and what "positives" he had shared about him. "I only vaguely remember," he wrote back. "I talked about his amazing ability as a truck driver ... He had an amazing ability as a mechanic as well. He also had lost a finger as a boy when his sister chased him with an old-fashioned barrel lawnmower. He must have teased her so much that she chased him with the mower, he accidentally fell and she ran over his hand, severing his finger. He had a party trick of being able to dent cans of food by smashing them over the stump of his missing finger. He was also a good storyteller with a strong imagination."

Brett's brother Adam attended both services, but Brett can't recall if his mother and sister did. His father's ashes were interned beside Brett's grandmother's grave, in the same cemetery that Brett had once slept in as a young man.

—

Aaron Johnstone was only a teenager when his path crossed Brett's, but he was already a damaged and dangerous young man. In 1998, Johnstone was seventeen, the son of a long-vanished father and victim of sexual abuse. He became a ward of the state at twelve and left school at fourteen, having already developed a ruinous addiction to drink and drugs. In time, if not already, he would form a "polysubstance dependence" on cannabis, alcohol, amphetamines, benzos and solvents.

On 19 June 1998, Johnstone was a resident of supervised community housing for youths in Dandenong. Brett and his partner were on patrol when they received the call: a young man, armed with a knife, was "going berserk" on the premises. He had threatened to kill four children, other residents of the home, who had locked themselves in a room. Brett took the job and requested backup.

It was a cold, misty night. They parked their patrol car across the road. From there, they could hear Johnstone screaming and the sounds of what they assumed to be the smashing of furniture.

The officers paced down the home's driveway, which stretched to the rear of the property. As they did, the supervising manager ran past them without stopping, screaming that Johnstone was trying to kill everyone and that "No money is worth this!"

The children were inside, now alone with Johnstone.

There was a grassed yard at the back of the building, and stairs leading up to glass sliding doors. From the yard, the officers could see into the home. Johnstone was holding a knife in one hand and a fire extinguisher in the other, and was using the extinguisher to trash the walls and furniture. They then saw Johnstone overturn the kitchen's oven – they didn't know it at the time, but in doing so, he had ruptured the gas pipes.

Brett saw how confined the space upstairs was. Such confinement is dangerous – it badly diminishes police control. In volatile circumstances with weapons involved, you want some distance. They requested backup again, were told none was available, and sought to distract Johnstone – they tried to coax him outside, away from the children. "There was no conversation between [my partner] and I," Brett said. "We didn't look at each other – we didn't need to. We were experienced policemen. After watching the male for a short time, he started to walk back in towards the interior of the house. Knowing there were children trapped somewhere in the house, this was the last thing we wanted. I immediately yelled to the male, using my booming military voice, for him to drop the knife and to come outside."

They now had Johnstone's attention, and they needed to keep it, to buy the children time. With the fire extinguisher, Johnstone smashed the door's glass panels, then hurled shards of glass at the officers while promising to kill them. "He yelled in detail how he was going to gut us and all the other ways he could kill us with the knife."

Johnstone now stepped outside, onto the landing. The officers were at the bottom of the stairs, perhaps ten steps away. Johnstone was approaching with the knife, still promising to slaughter them. Brett's partner removed his capsicum spray – which Brett, based on his experience with the wildly drug-affected, thought would be ineffectual. Brett drew his gun and, per his training, aimed it at the centre of Johnstone's chest.

"In my mind, I realised that if he lunged at us, I would only get the one chance to stop him before he would be all over us with the knife," Brett said. "[We were both] yelling repeatedly for all our worth at the male to stop, to drop the knife. All the while he advanced towards us while screaming back at us that he was going to kill us. As he advanced on us, I began to pull back on my trigger. Everything seemed to be in slow motion. The hammer of the firearm was almost all the way to the rear of the gun. I would only get one shot. If I didn't stop him, we would die."

Brett was now prepared to kill a man. Was, in fact, very close to killing him. He can recall precisely the weight of the gun, the feeling of the trigger. The moment – the images, the physical sensations, the emotion – are crystallised.

But what happened next confused him. With his gun trained on Johnstone, Brett could see, peripherally, his partner put away his capsicum spray and draw his retractable baton. Johnstone was now rushing down the stairs, and Brett's partner flicked the baton to extend it. But he lost control, and the baton flew from his hand.

"What happened next haunts me to this day," Brett said. "My partner rushed forward in front of my firearm to retrieve his baton. The hammer of my firearm was all the way back, as I was taking the shot to stop the charging male, who was now only three steps away and rushing at us with the knife raised in his hands. As [my partner] moved forward to retrieve his baton, he lost his footing and slipped on the damp grass. He fell face down at the bottom step, right in front of the male. The male, with the knife raised high, charged down in a stabbing motion at [him]."

Brett, losing his aim and incapable of recovering a safe shot, threw himself at Johnstone to thwart the stabbing of his partner. He expected to feel the blade as he did so – but somehow escaped it.

Johnstone recovered his footing and ran back upstairs. Inside, another flight of stairs led upstairs to the children's bedroom. Brett knew he had to stop Johnstone's second ascent. He gave chase, into the house, and then up the second flight, while desperately trying to re-holster his gun.

Brett caught Johnstone's ankles and pulled, tripping him. The two men wrestled, Brett trying to avoid the flashing knife. Brett could smell the escaped gas from the kitchen, combined with the smell of alcohol and petrol on Johnstone.

By now, Brett's partner had caught up. "I was struggling to hold the male when [my partner] took him in a headlock with his right arm ... In horror, I watched as the male took [my partner] in a headlock of his own ... [My partner] again lost his footing on the stairs and fell heavily with the male over him. I watched as the male raised and brought his right arm all the way back. I watched as, with full force, he thrust the knife towards the upper ribs of [my partner]. I lunged through the banisters and with both hands I grabbed the wrist of the male's hand holding the knife, and with all my strength stopped the point of the knife – perhaps only a centimetre away from entering [my partner's] ribs. By this time there were no holds barred, so I dragged the male's knife hand through the banisters, where I was fully prepared to break his arm if needed to get him to release his grip on the knife. He managed to drag the knife across the top of my hand before I got him to drop the knife, but I received only superficial cuts."

At last, they had him.

—

Johnstone was convicted of unlawful assault and property damage but was not imprisoned. Later, he would keep acquiring similar convictions – more than two dozen of them. His drinking reached implausible quantities – a daily slab of beer and bottle of vodka – and there were several admissions to psych wards. In 2006, after a night of heavy drinking with his friend and housemate, Phillip Higgins, Johnstone again became murderously enraged – because, he would later tell police, Higgins had sexually propositioned him. Higgins was much older, smaller and weaker than Johnstone and never stood a chance. Johnstone beat him with his fists and with a chair and stomped on him when he fell. Higgins's jaw was broken, as were six ribs and a bone in his neck. One of his teeth would later be found inside his punctured lung. As Higgins lay on the floor spitting blood, Johnstone seized a heavy concrete sculpture of a platypus and crushed his friend's skull with it.

Johnstone was convicted of Higgins's murder twice, after a retrial in 2011. "I believe that if your problems with alcohol are not addressed, you are highly likely to relapse into violent offending," the judge said at sentencing. "Indeed, you will have real difficulties in complying with the conditions of any parole which you may be granted. You will have to take steps to confront the damage the grog has already done to you and caused you to do to others. Unless you learn to control your drinking, and, in turn, manage your anger, your future is a very bleak one."

—

There is, of course, a difference between something happening and not happening – but that difference, as far as the nervous system is concerned, is not as great as you might think. This was true for Peter James, when he imagined the death of newly born Sonny Day in the plane. For Brett, his nervous system hangs on three "what ifs?" – three alternative realities whose consequences he so intensely imagined, it's *almost* as if they happened.

The first is the shooting of Johnstone. The second is the accidental shooting of his partner, as he leapt into Brett's firing line. Brett played both scenarios – firing a bullet into Johnstone's chest, or into the back of his colleague's head – obsessively in his mind, and his nervous system was distressingly animated each time.

The final scenario was his own death – of fatally absorbing Johnstone's knife when Johnstone rushed him. "I drove home [that evening] trying to process all that had happened," Brett said. "This had been too close. This incident where I had pulled my firearm to protect my life and others was just one of many over the years. There were many instances where an offender having pointed a firearm at me or charged at me with a knife resulted in me needing to raise my firearm. Fortunately, I personally have not taken that final action of shooting someone. However, I am still haunted by these incidents. I lay awake at night feeling sick at how close I had come to taking someone's life or perhaps losing my own."

The obscenity of Johnstone's later crime reanimated that earlier evening at the care home. It confirmed for Brett how dangerous the man was and how close someone had come to dying that night. Johnstone had been a bomb that was never defused.

—

They received the call in their patrol car, but they weren't properly equipped for it. Brett and his new, probationary partner were on their way to the station to help mediate some conflict resolution: an ill-tempered colleague had sworn at a teenage girl, and now her mother wanted an apology.

But before they got there, word came through: a train driver thought he might have hit someone. He wasn't certain, and he hoped he was wrong, but it sure felt like it. And so, the train was stopped on the tracks, not far from the suspected collision, and the driver was instructed to remain in his seat until investigators arrived. The passengers remained fixed in theirs too.

Brett and his partner's job now was to search for the potential body, along the pitch-dark tracks. They didn't have proper flashlights, so illuminated their way with the modest beam of Brett's keyring torch. They could see the silhouettes of trees, and the outline of the train a few hundred metres away. Brett assumed that the body, if there was a body, would be in this direction, and they made their way slowly.

Everything was quiet, and then there it was. Or there they were, the pieces. A head, some limbs, a burst torso. They could feel the warmth of the body drifting up from the tracks. They could smell the blood, like raw steak. They realised they'd stepped on body parts. The feet were found later, a hundred metres or so away.

Brett called it in, and their job now was to stay where they were. He could tell that his partner wasn't doing well: he looked nauseous, overwhelmed. And so, Brett sought to relieve his anguish by singing to him: The Wiggles' "Fruit Salad". There was no response from his partner, a good sign that Brett should have ceased his maladroit humour, but Brett persisted. He suggested they should have picked up some bread from the local bakery to better mop up the blood, and then he sang another Wiggles song about mashed potato. His partner was appalled.

"I was trying to ease his pain, but he never spoke to me again. He probably thought I was the biggest arsehole in the world. I thought he was the biggest sook in the world."

—

I wondered if Brett wasn't also trying to induct his partner into a world where a calloused familiarity with the obscene was not only necessary but expressed with cowboy puerility. In my experience, coppers have both a fierce belief in the usefulness of black humour and a zealous sense of entitlement to its use. And with good reason. In a profession that exposes its members to macabre destructions, they don't appreciate outsiders policing their humour.

But Brett's story badly jarred me. Not only for what he had said, but for his inability or reluctance to see how his puerility had aggravated his inexperienced partner. The value of black humour surely depends upon its reception. In this case, it evidently did not achieve its stated goal of relieving the pain of Brett's stricken partner – arguably, it made it worse. Brett had an exaggerated faith in the therapeutic value of his humour, and he misread the moment. His ear failed him.

As we've seen, Brett has an ambivalent relationship with the idea of compassion. Maintaining compassion and toughness in perfect equilibrium was often impossible, and the two values anxiously circled each other in Brett's world view. The deprivations of his childhood may have encouraged empathy with the public, but he had also been programmed for toughness and rigidity.

While telling the story of the train suicide, Brett abruptly returned to a scene from his basic army training. They were performing drills on the hot, black tarmac. The sun was merciless. Some of the recruits fainted from the heat. Another vomited. The hard-arsed corporal marched over, stuck his finger into the puddle of sick, and licked it. "Did I give you permission to vomit, son?!" That was how it was. That's how the wheat was separated from the chaff. And after initially thinking that he wasn't smart enough or tough enough to survive basic training, Brett was told that he was, in fact, good enough. Having overcome his insecurity and found competency within a hallowed tribe, it was unlikely that he would now question its values. He was determined to "make something of himself", to correct for his poisoned self-esteem, and he chose vocations in which toughness was thought sacred. To do his job, to be *seen* to be doing his job, and to *be seen by himself* to be doing his job, he would sometimes have to contradict other instincts and other lessons he had learnt on the beaches of Surfers Paradise and in the orphanage. Toughness and compassion were not always mutually exclusive. But sometimes they were.

–

PTSD means having a nervous system that's too easily aroused. A burst balloon can excite a spasm of anxiety and release a flood of adrenaline. Your amygdala, your brain's ancient lighthouse keeper and surveyor of danger, loses its powers of discrimination. It's as though there's a splinter lodged in your mind. Preoccupied with unprocessed memories and therefore permanently primed, the amygdala can no longer distinguish between triviality and danger. Which is why, at my daughter's fifth birthday, I feared the happy string of balloons decorating her party room – and why I insisted that I pop them afterwards. At least I was in control then. In popping the balloons myself, I was killing the chance of being surprised.

It's exhausting. Typically, the human body is not frequently soaked in adrenaline or other stress hormones. Their release usually corresponds to an external threat that would justify them – a danger against which the flight-or-fight instinct might be usefully animated. But with PTSD, it happens *constantly*, and the subtler, analytical departments of the mind defer entirely to the reptilian one.

There's also a wicked shingling of symptoms: the exhaustion of constant adrenal shocks, combined with the exhaustion of having your sleep repeatedly spiked by nightmares, corrodes your resilience. Ordinary, everyday stresses – things you've spent a lifetime acquitting well and without trouble – get harder. Scarier. And then follows another degradation: faith in yourself. Faith that you can keep your shit together.

It was worse for Brett. His nervous system was permanently electrified. He experienced constant surges of adrenaline and sought to recklessly purge them. Sometimes, he'd place himself in a holding cell with a violent, drug-addled suspect and just sit there. He was looking for a fight – or, if not a fight, at least some external circumstance that might correspond with his intolerably high levels of anxiety and adrenaline. To sit with an electrified nervous system with no correspondent external reality is strangely, almost ineffably painful – so Brett went looking for situations that would justify or relieve it.

Come fucking fight me. Let me taste danger, risk. You may see this as toxic bravura, and unprofessional, and it's certainly at least one of those things. But I can understand the purgatorial desire – the need to find a circumstance that can make sense of, and even make useful, the sparks of a damaged nervous system. Without one, the disconnect between your nervous system and your environment can be distressingly jarring.

So, Brett went hunting for crooks. And he became angry. *Very* angry. The job had naturally encouraged his disgust and sharpened his anger, but the righteousness of that anger was also bound up with his identity; he accepted it as proof of his legitimacy as a member of the police tribe.

"The drug dealers, the heavy crooks, feared me," Brett said. "Feared me terribly. If I pulled up and they saw me in the divvy van, you'd see them run. We're chasing one crook, my partner and I, through this park. They saw me at the top of the hill, and these two were having a nice picnic and jumped up and threw themselves in the river to get to the other side, to get away from me. The ferocity and the hate we cannot mention here. We cannot mention here."

"Did the hate overwhelm you?" I asked him.

"I don't know what you mean by 'overwhelm'."

"Did it drown out other feelings, I guess – a sense of perspective, prudence, compassion? Hate has that capacity – to drown out all other things."

"Yes, absolutely."

Brett saw things, repeatedly, that sickened him. "I developed an absolute – and it almost goes against all my nature and personality – but for drug addicts in particular, I developed an absolute hate," he said. "The elderly people and the children that were traumatised, the families that were broken, this was constant – 99 per cent of the work was drug-related at St Kilda or Dandenong, and when I did undercover work at Frankston, it was drugs. You'd find little eighteen-month-old babies crawling down the street, and find where they live, and you go in, and it would be squalor and syringes all over the floor."

Brett had seen this too many times. His disgust and sorrow would yield to rage. I'm not sure Brett knows where, exactly, professional diligence ended and darkly ungovernable emotion began. I can't say, either. But his disgust and sorrow at seeing babies crawling the street alone were natural. His rage, too. Just as Peter James's impulse to kick the corpse of the man who'd shot his own baby – the baby Peter was carrying – seems natural, at the same time as it is undeniably unprofessional.

If we accept that rage and disgust are unprofessional and should not be expressed indiscriminately, we may also have to accept that for first responders, professionalism may require a degree of numbness and detachment, a forgetting of the more idealistic version of themselves who signed up for the gig. And if we accept that, then we might assume that moral injury and self-alienation are inescapable.

–

One day in late 2013, while I was working for the chief commissioner of Victoria Police, I saw a despondent – perhaps tearful – Detective Senior Sergeant Ron Iddles enter the chief's office and close the door.

Iddles was professionally admired – a veteran homicide investigator and perhaps the state's most recognisable officer. A year earlier, he had successfully led the high-profile investigation of Jill Meagher's murder. But on the day I saw him head into the chief commissioner's office, Iddles himself had made front-page news and was the subject of the morning's talkback radio programs. Many – including the state's premier – thought that he'd disgraced both the police force and the memory of Meagher.

Iddles, while periodically suffering his own trauma and exhaustion, was also impressively untiring. When not investigating murders, he often spoke publicly – driven, I believe, not by ego (which can afflict detectives) but by a desire to share with the public both the technical realities and methods of police work and the moral weight of crimes that the public and media too often treat as macabre entertainments.

In the week before Iddles entered the chief's office, he had given a public presentation about his work, including the Jill Meagher investigation. The event was a charity fundraiser: audience members paid to attend, but Iddles, as always, did not accept a speaking fee. He had become something of a touring preacher – sermonising about the work of homicide detectives and about the ghosts they found along the way. He invited audiences to remember the souls of murder victims and the souls of those who investigated their deaths.

Iddles had given the same presentation before, and it included – briefly – a picture of Jill Meagher in her shallow grave. Crucially, Iddles had sought permission from Meagher's family to show the image, and permission was given. After the presentation, two people complained. From there, the presentation quickly attracted media interest and the weight of scandal. The premier at the time said, "When I heard about this yesterday afternoon, I was sickened, I was shocked, and immediately my heart went out to the Meagher family." An acting deputy commissioner of Victoria Police publicly apologised to the public and to Meagher's family, implying (wrongly) that they had not consented and had taken offence, and described the presentation as an unfortunate lapse of judgement by Iddles.

Once a certain threshold had been crossed – once it seemed established in the public conversation that Iddles's presentation was both rogue and insensitive – no argument was offered and no defence of Iddles was made. Instead, the weight of "public feeling" was anxiously deferred to. The worst characterisation of the event was accepted as the only one. No one seemed to know or care that Iddles had the full support of Meagher's family, and his reputation was smeared.

I was angered at the time and respectfully said as much to the acting deputy commissioner – the man who'd made the public apology and a man I very much liked. Nonetheless, I felt that Iddles had been abandoned and that crude, incomplete assumptions had been left unchallenged.

No one wants vain, insensitive detectives boastfully sharing their "war stories" in public, and certainly not when the stories involve rape and murder. But that's not what happened here. Iddles was a gifted detective and a serious man. He was also haunted. He'd joined Victoria Police in 1980 and left nine years later, burnt out. He went and drove trucks, before re-entering the force a few years later and beginning again at the rank of constable. Later, when he had time off, he'd find peace, or something close to it, by driving interstate coaches. Here was a man earnestly trying to show the soul of police work – practically and spiritually. The hard work and the squalor. The methods and the obscenity. *Here is the job*, he was saying. *Please recognise the dead souls and the work of finding their killers. Please see what we see and do.*

I appreciate this isn't a popular view, and perhaps it's instinctively self-serving, too: for what else is this book but my asking you to contemplate the work and its profound costs? Which might explain my sympathy for something broadly considered ill-judged or even repulsive at the time, and something which no one I've spoken to since can support.

—

I'm aware of the risk, as I write this book, of numbing you, the reader, with a repetitive anthology of carnage. I'm sensitive to leavening it, truncating it, and removing things altogether. I'm sensitive to your notional appetites and stamina, as I'm sensitive to the elements of crafting a book – of building and releasing tension, for example, but also of handling macabre material in a manner that neither corrupts it, nor alienates you. There's manipulation, in other words, a manipulation that I hope remains faithful to the realities it describes and yet retains your interest – because, after a time, those dead souls become just dull words, right?

But this book necessarily describes a procession of death and misery; of blood and flayed flesh; and of the fluctuating sense of competency and guilty ineptitude that those responding to it feel – necessarily, because the fact of its seeming endlessness is a critical point for the very subjects of this book.

So for you, the reader, I can leaven, truncate, cut. I can introduce passages, like this one, that offer some small respite. Brett couldn't.

His breaking point – if there was such a neatly discrete moment – followed an accumulation of stress. He went to work and took the calls. Sometimes there were good shifts; sometimes there were three, four, five separate fatalities in eight hours. Death could seem endless.

There was the time when he attended a road crash and a motorcyclist had been literally flattened yet had somehow remained alive. The paramedic who arrived was paralysed by what he saw; Brett assumed he was experiencing a nervous breakdown and helped him back to the cabin of his ambulance. Or the time he was called to a hairdresser's salon where a client was experiencing a fatal asthma attack, and Brett held the man as he died. Or the industrial accidents that mangled bodies in unthinkable ways, or the young girls dead in alleyways with needles in their arms, or the countless suicides and SIDS deaths and drownings. Once, Brett hugged the corpse of a teenager he knew and was reprimanded for his unprofessionalism.

"Not every shift was like that," Brett said. "But sometimes you see just way too much, too often. Sometimes, in a couple of weeks, you're just going from one death to another, and they might not be gruesome – they might be just heart attacks. But you almost feel that all you're doing is being around dead people all the time. It feels like it's more normal to be dead than alive."

One of Brett's "war stories" echoed Mike Ryan's framework: high demand, low control, low predictability.

It was 17 June 2002. Brett was out in the divisional van with a fresh, trainee officer. Within minutes of starting their patrol, their radio became busy with alerts about a multi-vehicle accident on the Monash Freeway. The trainee asked if they could attend – he'd not yet seen a traffic accident and wanted to learn how police responded.

Brett was reluctant – they were on divisional van duties, and the radio had confirmed that specialist traffic management units were already attending. But he agreed, thinking that if something else came up they could easily divert themselves.

At the scene, they found a hellscape. Several trucks and many more cars were twisted and entangled, their dead occupants hanging from windows. The dying were splayed on the road; the badly injured were crawling across it. Brett called for more ambulances, the fire brigade, even the SES – and then he noticed his junior partner entering shock. "He had turned as white as white can be," Brett said. "He appeared to start to faint, and I immediately took hold of him and assisted him to the bushes at the side of the freeway."

Brett left him there and returned to a scene that was much bloodier and more chaotic than he'd anticipated.

"There was a man staggering and falling across the freeway towards me," he said. "He was covered in blood. His collarbone was clearly broken, with his arm hanging in the most unusual manner as he tried to support it with his other arm. His face was unrecognisable due to the blood streaming down his face. I was almost overwhelmed by the scale of the situation. There were so many people seriously injured. Blood was flowing from so many. [There were] broken bones and unconscious, maimed bodies. I felt like I was in a war zone. The magnitude of this accident felt impossible to control or comprehend. I felt the fear of being helpless."

But then, Brett said, a feeling of calm suddenly came over him, followed by clarity and efficiency. He said his military training, and whatever instincts he'd absorbed after eleven years in the police force, assumed primacy. "My mind seemed to change gear," he said. "I immediately set up a triage post, and I recruited the uninjured to assist me with the injured. I was able to take charge without faltering."

It was chaotic. As well as the gravely injured, one of the trucks was carrying a great volume of industrial acid. The man Brett saw staggering across the freeway was subsequently hit by a car. A truck driver, whose vehicle was untouched by the pile-up, left his cabin and was also struck by a passing car.

Obviously, the scene had not been contained. Brett received a call requesting he take charge as forward commander of the incident. He ordered the closure of the Monash Freeway. He took charge, as he'd been instructed to. But he also thought: *My God, what fucking next?*

He was burnt out. "Later in my career, my nerves and strength seemed to fail me," he said. "I had seen too much and witnessed such horror. At times during large, tense and life-threatening situations, I developed involuntary shakes. On the surface I was rock solid. A tower of strength and in charge. A beacon of control. However, my hands or my leg would shake uncontrollably. Fortunately, I was always able to hide this by putting my hand in my pocket or under my uniform. At times I thought my quivering voice may have given me away. No one seemed to suspect that somewhere, at some time, I got broken."

—

Brett would come to feel that death was everywhere, that he lived inside death, that everyone he spoke to was already dead. This wasn't poetic melancholy, or grim detachment, but a genuinely held and very literal delusion: *that everyone he saw was dead.*

"I remember when it began," he told me. "It began after an industrial fatality. Everyone was dead. You'd be sitting here talking to me as you are now, and I'd be looking at a dead person that was talking. That lasted for years. I don't know how to – I don't know the psychology of it. But everyone was walking around, dead."

By now, in the early 2000s, Brett was also experiencing the arrows of intrusive memories. Lots of them, and all the time. He had acquired so many traumatic memories, each one piercing when they arrived unbidden, that he developed his own metaphor for his mind: it was a giant warehouse containing aisles upon aisles of filing cabinets, each stuffed with obscene images, that some cruel and independent power would randomly open and expose to him. *Here, Brett – remember this?*

Brett became sick – really sick. He first noticed that something was wrong after driving back to the station after he'd taken photos of a particularly nasty industrial accident. "Was something wrong with my judgement and reflexes?" he said. "I first noticed it when I was driving on a long, straight stretch of road. It was early morning. It was clear, with little traffic. Yet I saw a car approaching a stop sign leading onto the road I was on. This car was hundreds of metres in front of me and had cautiously pulled up at the stop sign. For some reason I found myself slamming on the brakes. I was overreacting, being overcautious. I noted that I wasn't able to drive faster than walking speed. I crawled into the station and resumed making my cup of tea."

The symptoms were classic. His hands trembled. He wept spontaneously. He feared the work he once loved and which had come to singularly define him; some days, he'd vomit on his way there. His anxiety was extreme and relentless. It felt like an orchestral crescendo in his head that never ended – it would just infinitely climb in pitch. He was exhausted and irritable. He couldn't sleep. He was losing his sense of control and perspective. He experienced depression and idly thought of suicide. He questioned his capacity for love and doubted his professional competency and judgement.

But when all this became apparent, when the symptoms he thought he was concealing so well finally became obvious to others, he "fought tooth and nail" to keep his job. After all, "I wasn't a man or a human being," he said. "I was a police officer." His entire identity depended upon this job. If he wasn't a police officer, he didn't quite know who he was – perhaps just more of the world's damaged refuse.

One day, in 2008, Brett was called by the police medical officer. They told him he could no longer be out on the streets, but suggested a desk job could be arranged instead. "You don't realise how sick you are," they said. Brett disagreed and defiantly went doctor shopping, securing medical certificates testifying to his health. This prolonged his service, but only by a few months.

He was sick – but he was also in denial. One day, Brett returned to the station with two burglary suspects, even though he was not rostered for operational duty. Regardless, he was pleased with himself and intended to interview them. But the station's senior sergeant called him over, and she wasn't pleased. "She's looking at me with her arms crossed," he said. "'Brett, come and talk to me,' she said. And in the hallway there, she asked me for the keys to the divvy van. I gave her the keys, and then her voice changed. She's very hesitant. And she said, 'Would you please give me your firearm.' It hit hard. Her first words to me were, 'You can't be here.' She sounded scared. And I'm thinking: 'Where to from here?' because I couldn't think of being anything else but a police officer."

I was struck by Brett's saying that his senior sergeant seemed scared. Was he so sick, and so removed from self-understanding, that his colleagues thought he was a threat?

"I knew that a lot was wrong, and had been for years," he said. "But I was very protective of other police. There's some dickhead police out there, but I'd protect them with my life. So I was never a threat to another police officer. But the way she sounded, sounded awful." His sergeant's voice, and her order to surrender his firearm, were humiliating. Brett now saw his own sickness head-on. The end had come.

In 2008, Brett was placed on indefinite medical leave pending examination. That came more than a year later, in October 2009, when he was examined by several doctors. The police medical officer would confirm his medical retirement: "I do believe that Brett's major depressive disorder and post-traumatic stress disorder are resulting from traumatic events he had been involved in as a police officer over the years," their report read. "I do not believe Brett is capable of returning to the duties of a police officer because if they traumatise him his mental state may deteriorate further. I do not believe that he would be able to occupy that role at any stage in the future."

To be asked to surrender the tools of his job – the glorified and deadly tools that signified an exalted authority – was diminishing enough. But with medical retirement came an empty room, and silence. Brett now experienced the dissolution of his identity, and the jagged discrepancy between a screamingly adrenalised inner life and the mocking torpor of retirement. He was not yet fifty.

"They told me I'll be on medication for the rest of my life," he said. "This is the final briefing from the police medical officer. You will have to take medication the rest of your life. Antidepressants, antipsychotics, a whole magnitude of medications for life. I was already anti-drug. I wouldn't even take a Panadol, because I hated drug addicts so much. And now I'm told I'll be on all this for the rest of my life.

"And they say: 'Now, Brett, find a quiet room in your house and never leave it for the rest of your life. If you leave your house, you'll probably become overwhelmed. Don't leave your house, because you might have to be hospitalised. See you later.' So, I went home. And it was the worst thing. I was in my lounge room. It's all quiet, and there's nothing to do, and it's like just taking me out of a battlefield of twenty years of fighting and plonking me in a quiet room. No wonder so many people hang themselves. It's the worst possible thing you can do to somebody. Your adrenaline's still going, your mind's still going, and here you are in a quiet room with no release, no anything. It was a tough few years going through that."

Given Brett's own admissions, I'm sure he'll accept my view that he should have been operationally retired – indeed, should have been much sooner than he was. But the question of transition remains: how best to use the retired talents of those for whom the job has been existentially defining? Operational retirement may be necessary, but this need not mean automatic eviction from the fraternity that has defined the retiring officer. In Brett's case, he was an accomplished horseman, and he wonders if he could have been deployed as a trainer in the mounted branch. As a boy in the orphanage, he had once dreamt of joining the cavalry. Such an appointment might have offered a satisfying closing of a circle.

No such appointment was offered. But then, Brett said, he might not have been the most pleasant colleague during his last few years in the force.

—

Brett had assumed a role, against great odds, that repaired his self-esteem, rewarded his devotion and complemented his faith in authority. He had found a vocation that partially vanquished the suspicions he held about himself, by seeming to confirm him as a decent, courageous and influential member of society. And so his pride and sense of identity were forged – but they were forged in a very hot oven, and eventually the heat would break him again.

I once knew a former detective who, after a long career investigating murders, retired to the country, where he worked on his small boat and went fishing whenever he desired. After decades of heavy public service, he could retreat without regret to years of fishing on languid waters in a boat he periodically re-seals and touches with paint. He was a sweet man, and while I wondered what baggage he might be taking with him into these years of leisure, the arrangement seemed right. I hoped he might commit his attention to tides and bait and the cooking of the day's catch for his wife. I hoped the gentleness of these days might feel earnt and natural, and that he would enjoy them without intrusive memories or guilt.

It wasn't this way for Brett. He couldn't retreat into years of leisure. He still wants to be defined by public service. And I think he still wants the specific pride and personal definition that his old job gave him.

And so, he has continued to hold his hand to the flame. He speaks at RSL clubs, where his phone number is passed between members. He once told me he'd been on the phone all night, talking another ex-cop down from the ledge of suicide. He also told me that he'd cut down the body of a neighbour who had hung himself. Another time, we postponed a conversation after he told me: "I have been tied up this week with an unusually complex suicide intervention."

I wasn't sure what to make of this. Brett had been removed from the job, but he still wanted to save souls. He told me about that intervention, involving a long-retired cop who had tried to kill himself in the shed he was living in. It was an overdose, and the man had been taken to hospital but then defiantly left. A neighbour called Brett, assuming the man had returned home "to finish the job".

"I was able to step in gently and say, 'How about we go for a coffee at a local café?'" Brett said. "My reasoning was, it's a public place. It's under cameras. We had lunch together for a couple of hours. And I listened to him, and we shared some old war stories and had a bit of a laugh. We spoke about the trauma of the job, but he said that he was never traumatised – it was water off a duck's back, were his words. But then he would go into some quite gruesome stuff that we would deal with. And then, when I thought it was the right time, I said, 'Look, we need to go back to the hospital.'"

Brett told me about several interventions like this. The day before one of our interviews, he later said, he'd spent the morning in his backyard with several cups of tea, "trying to process it all and get some energy back".

After his second divorce, Brett still has his children if not a marriage. He speaks of them often and describes things he has planned for them or things they've done in the past: fireworks, barbecues, road trips.

There's the local RSL, and he's also in contact with ex-police who share his injuries. He sits on three committees at a local hospital, one of which he conducts safety audits for. He visits elderly patients with little or no family. Within these networks, Brett has developed a reputation for being someone you can call in a crisis. I suspect he couldn't have it any other way.

Brett's still tethered to his past, and the sense of self that the old job gave him. He's still giving himself, too, but I can't say exactly what the cost is. But I think I can say this: that Brett's childhood funnelled him towards public service, where he found great conviction and purpose before finding more trauma. But despite the nightmares, the waking one is worse: of being stripped of his purpose and of the glory of a job that, for a time, so gloriously defied what he had long assumed to be the world's contempt for his prospects. That's a hard thing to lose – the thing that defied the worst things you think about yourself. And so, for now, Brett finds purpose as a freelancing volunteer, still communing with the dark.

3

The Firie

TARA LAL

"I wanted to help people, for that was what gave me a sense of self-worth."

Tara was thirteen when she watched her mother's coffin pass through the curtain. She wondered why no one was stopping it from entering the flames. She didn't want to let her go.

As the coffin crossed its final threshold, Tara winced as she remembered her embarrassment about her mother's wig when the two were out in public. Her mother, Bridget, was gone now, and Tara's guilt could never be confessed to the person she most wanted to confess it to.

It was 1984, and Tara's family – her father Shivaji and her

older siblings Adam and Jo – were attending their mother's funeral service in the same North London church where her parents were married eighteen years before. Bridget had been diagnosed with cancer five years earlier. Tara remembered being called to her mother's bedside and being told "I think I'm dying – I don't want to leave you." She remembered her mother's yellow skin and straw-like hair. Her mother was fifty-one years old when she died.

—

Two decades later, in Sydney in 2005, Tara was accepted into the NSW Fire Brigade's training college. A few weeks into a sixteen-week course, she was about to enter the "hot cell" – a smoky and intensely heated metallic maze that she would have to navigate blindfolded while wearing protective gear and a heavy breathing kit. Recruits were warned not to drink booze or exercise too vigorously in the days beforehand, given the litres of sweat they would release in the "cell". Tara would later remove her boots and pour the stuff out like she was tipping a jug of beer.

Such was the thickness of her protective clothing, Tara was already overheating before she entered the maze. The compressed-air tanks on her back had clownishly realigned her centre of balance. To succeed, she and her partner would have to overcome their imbalance, blindness and fear.

Tara entered first, her partner close behind her. The heavy metal door shut behind them, and the heat was stunning. It was a "left-hand search", meaning the two would navigate by keeping their left hands on the nearest wall of the maze, collect the dummy casualty and return by using their right hands along the same wall. The wall was meant to orient them amid their blindness and panic.

But Tara fumbled, becoming unsure in the hot, smoky darkness. She felt for an opening, then radioed her partner that she could not find a path forward. Keep trying, he told her.

And she did. But she became even more lost. Somehow, she found herself beneath the maze – a fact irritably relayed to her by the instructor, who was watching their progress from inside the labyrinth via thermal-imaging cameras. And that was it. They were called back, the exercise over. Panting, they pushed the door open and were received by an unimpressed instructor.

"Congratulations," he told Tara. "You've just killed yourself, your partner and your victim."

Tara went home to her apartment. Here it was again, she thought: the funk of fear and shame. She had a long and intense relationship with shame, and she wondered if she was strong enough to prevail: she'd have to enter the maze again tomorrow.

She was anxious about going back in, but more anxious about failing the test again and what such a failure would mean for the ideas she held about her resilience and fitness for the job. She had sought a tough and purposeful vocation. If she failed this test, she was sure her very self-conception would fail too.

They were instructed to retrieve the "casualty" – a 75-kilogram dummy – from within the hot, smoky and claustrophobic maze. Tara was no less fearful than she had been the day before, but this time she focused on the physical: her hands, her orientation and then, when they found the dummy, hauling it down from its ledge.

They successfully performed the rescue. Within two months, Tara graduated as a firefighter and was posted to Sydney's busiest station.

–

Tara's colleagues included Spy, Boaty and Normy. There was also Digby and Big Gez. Tara was The Bear, so-called because she was grumpy when the bells woke her. You don't choose your nickname, and she didn't mind hers. In fact, for a long time, she loved station culture: the blokey banter, the irreverence, the collegial familiarity. It felt like another family, and she didn't mind the great preponderance of men. She was the station's only woman. Today, women comprise about 15 per cent of the NSW fire service. When Tara joined, it was around 5 per cent.

She won arm wrestles in the mess room. As the junior member, she was saddled with the heavy "goat bag" – the one containing the high-rise kit. She was mocked good-naturedly when, woken one evening by the bells, she hurriedly dressed and slid down the nearest pole, only to realise that her yellow bedsheet had somehow caught in her pants and now trailed behind her like a large security blanket. For a moment there, her nickname almost changed to "Linus".

"There was a lot of humour," Tara said. "In my experience, the humour was not used against me or pointed towards me. It was a shared way of coping, and we laughed together. There weren't people laughing at me or using it as a form of bullying or harassment. I know that that does exist, and has existed for other female firefighters, most definitely. But from my own experiences, I didn't actually feel that. You know, the humour was actually an important part of being able to lighten the heaviness."

She told me about one job, a "red message" – a priority. She remembers fastening her safety harness in the truck as they sped towards the Maroubra Seals Club, and the excitement and sense of purpose she felt. The top floor of the club was ablaze, and a brief structural survey suggested the roof would likely collapse. Tara was part of a specialist truck – one equipped with an "aerial ladder" – and it was the first one there. They ran the hose up the ladder and Tara assessed the "monitor" – the high-capacity water jet. As Digby fixed the hose to the hydrant, then ran it through a separate truck's pump, Tara put on her breathing apparatus and harnessed herself to the ladder's cage.

They were ready. Tara raised the ladder to the top floor, where she could clearly see the fire. But it wasn't simply a matter of engaging the monitor and dousing the flames. She knew that the roof was badly compromised, and the weight of the water could trigger its collapse. Before she added to the roof's burden, she had to satisfy herself that her colleagues had left the building.

She received confirmation of this by radio, then felt the hose shiver with the coming water. It was dark, windy and smoky. She could see the glimmer of floating embers. She turned the monitor on, adjusting its spray for the wind. Soon, the fire was extinguished and the smoke cleared. There were no serious injuries. It was a job well done.

She enjoyed the thrill of competent camaraderie and the gratification of work that so obviously helped the public. But Tara was still dogged by wavering confidence. "Early on in my firefighting career, I felt insecure," Tara said. "[I worried] that I didn't know enough, and that probably stayed with me for most of my career."

Sometimes Tara went to jobs as the pump driver. It's a difficult role; the pump driver must engage the truck's pump, set up the hose, monitor most radio communication and find water. A city truck's water tank is limited, meant only as a stopgap. How long its water supply lasts will depend upon the pressure used and the size of the hose and tank, but typically you only have a few minutes. On most city blocks, a couple of feet below the road or footpath, fire hydrants have been installed. Usually, in metropolitan areas, they're no more than 100 metres apart and clearly visible. But not always. They might be obscured by grass or by an illegally parked car. If a hydrant can't be found nearby, several lengths of hose may be required to connect the truck's pump to a hydrant further up the street. This costs time.

One day, Tara could not find water. Her firies were waiting impatiently, using what they knew to be the last of the tank's supply. The situation was simple, Tara said: she needed to find water. If she didn't, "[people] can die and shit can happen".

The radio was busy too, and when a second pump driver arrived, the two of them conferred. Tara assumed from their conversation that he would take over the hydrant search while she ran radio co-ordination and managed the pump. But through either miscommunication or distraction, the second pump driver was in fact monitoring the deployment of a ladder, while Tara was busy with other duties. The most basic element of the job – finding water – had fallen between them.

Tara didn't realise this until she heard the urgent shouts of her colleagues. "A job can be chaos," Tara said. "You have all these plans in place, but it rarely runs smoothly. I could hear that the pump was running out. So I ran miles up the street and then ran three lengths of hose down to the pump. People are screaming, 'Get the water!'

"Nothing catastrophic happened on that job, but I crucified myself for it. I felt like I'd done a shit job. I crucified myself over and over. In my head, people were looking at me, thinking *Fuck, she's useless*. That's the narrative I tell myself. But then other times, people come up to me and say, 'Shit, you're such a good firie', and I think – *am I?*

"Growing up, I thought everything was my fault. I thought my dad's illness was my fault. That Dad was sick because of me. Rationally, many years later, I knew that wasn't the case. But I absorbed that. I embedded that thought process. I still apologise often for things that have nothing to do with me. It's an automatic response."

Tara has had a long relationship with shame. When she was eleven, she wrote in her diary: "Dad's depressed. I hate it when Dad's depressed because he's so quiet and I always think it's my fault."

—

All high-rise buildings are fitted with automatic fire alarms (AFAs) that, when triggered, alert the nearest fire station. Firies hate them. Notoriously fickle, they produce enormous numbers of false alarms. In 2023, Fire and Rescue NSW responded to roughly 50,000 alerts, only 2 per cent of which were real emergencies.

A fire crew will typically know it is a false alarm before they arrive, because the dispatch team will be quiet. A genuine fire would trigger not only an AFA but also a triple zero call from the public. So it was one evening in Darlinghurst, in central Sydney, as Tara and her colleagues raced to a residential tower – they were responding to an AFA, but there was no other sign of public distress.

But once they arrived, Tara could see smoke pouring from the eighth floor. It was a real job. Their breathing kits were already fixed to their backs, and they had their high-rise "goat bag" with them. They set up their hose on the floor below the fire. The radio was busy, the building's automated evacuation alert was blaring, and residents were making their exit.

When the hose was ready, the team headed to the eighth floor. The fire seemed contained to one apartment. "It's a residential building and the middle of the night," Tara said. "So you assume that it's occupied, and that you need to get in there quickly."

But there was a problem. Most doors open inwards and can be forced open by applying an axe with the firefighter's Halligan tool, a combination of pickaxe and crowbar. But this door opened outwards, and its cramped location at the end of a corridor restricted how much leverage they could apply. In such a situation, firefighters might use a hydraulic tool to force the door, but one hadn't arrived.

There was another complication. Once they opened the door, they knew the corridor would instantly fill with smoke. Anyone who hadn't yet evacuated would have to be ordered to stay inside their unit. That included the incident commander, who was without his breathing apparatus – it wasn't unusual for commanders to arrive at AFAs without them, if the comms team was quiet and a false alarm had been assumed.

Eventually, the team forced entry. Tara entered the dark, smoky apartment with her partner for a quick search and rescue operation. If there were people inside, their priority was finding and removing them.

Visibility was nil, and Tara quickly lost her partner. She was utterly disoriented. "Normally, you would try to stay connected to [your partner], but we kind of lost contact," Tara remembers. "It was the first time I didn't fucking know where I was. It's so disorientating. It's pitch black. You don't know the layout of the unit. We didn't have a thermal imaging camera with us. I remember that moment of thinking: *shit*."

Tara was comforted, however, by the absence of heat. This wasn't a raging inferno. Nor, it turned out, was the apartment occupied. Tara found the source of the fire, opened a window to ventilate the smoke and recovered her partner.

Catastrophe was averted, and the imagination's anxious conjuring was happily unfulfilled. But that sense of disorientation lingered with Tara. The sudden lack of control. It was a familiar feeling.

—

When Tara's mother lay dying, she wrote letters to her three children, which she intended to be read only after her death. Each letter was meant, of course, to comfort and guide them in the wake of her passing. But the letters were later compared by the children and found to express different expectations for each of them. To her son Adam, she wrote:

> I don't know when you will read this, but you are fifteen as I write it. I am very proud of you and love you dearly and want you to know that. You will have most of your life still before you and it makes me very sad to realize I have shared so little of it with you. I presume you will miss me, but once all of you have recovered from your sadness, I hope you will pick up the threads of your lives again, piece them together in a meaningful way and gradually, when the grieving is over, the happy memories will sustain you.
>
> You have a special place in my life, Adam. A mother's only son inevitably makes her proud and full of expectation and hope. We have tried as you know to give you the sort of education that we thought you could benefit from, but it has been difficult for me as you know I have a socialist philosophy and do not believe in an elitist society. On the other hand, I do believe that a chap's potential should be encouraged and

developed to the full and you have plenty of that. Diligence and single-mindedness and a sense of direction will, I am sure, achieve for you a university place. I'm sure that is your aim as well as Dad's and mine and of course whatever you do afterwards is up to you.

I have always nursed a dream that my son should go to Oxbridge, specifically, I think, because it is something in the family that nobody has yet achieved. Maybe you will be the first to do so! But wherever you go, enjoy your university days – alas Dad will find it hard financially but you will get a grant and you will simply have to live on it, but then lots of chaps do. Always in life, the more you put into it the more you will get out of it, and always remember that whatever you do, you are part of the community, the wider world, and every citizen has a responsibility toward that community, to care, to give and to take a share in responsibility for it. You will, I am sure, be able to help Dad a lot – he will need it. Jo will be able to cope herself, but Tara will need all of you. Do help each other all you can and try to see each other's needs. I have trusted Jo through her adolescence and I trust you too. Above all, Adam, be happy and fulfilled. Goodbye my son and good luck.

All my love,

Mum

Adam would later confide to Tara the weight of the letter: how specific their mother's dreams were and how incapable he felt of fulfilling them. Tara would come to realise the significance of this for her brother, but at the time she couldn't help but notice how much longer Adam's letter was and how much more expansive were the ambitions it expressed for him.

Tara's letter read:

> Tara, my love, I hope it will be a long, long time before you read this letter, but I wanted to write each of you a letter to keep for yourselves to remember your old mum. Darling, I do feel I have let you down so badly and have been able to share so little of your life with you. You will miss me – or I suppose you will – but when you have recovered from the initial shock and sadness I am sure you will all be able to help each other because I know how much you care for one another. Dad will, I know, need lots of help, but I know you will give him that help and give him lots of cuddles. I wanted so much to see you grow up, get married and have children – the things that any mother wants – but alas it has not been so. But whatever you do in life, darling, I want you first of all to be happy, secondly to lead a useful and caring life and thirdly to marry and have children eventually, because I know they will give you much pleasure in the way that you have all done for me.

Four years later, when the darkest shadow was cast again upon the family, Tara would painfully reconsider those letters. But at the time she clutched hers like a talisman. She had little else, and her father was melting.

Within days of his wife's death, Shivaji swung between euphoria and severe depression. Both extremes were disturbing.

In his most effusive states, he resembled a stranger, unable to acknowledge the death of his wife. In his depression, he could not even acknowledge his children. "I'm not sure he experienced grief," Tara said. "He experienced psychosis. I don't remember the grief. There were no real visual signs that he was grieving. In fact, in his psychosis it was like Mum's death was the best thing that ever happened. And that's really difficult in helping you process grief when you can't see your father grieving. I'm sure he felt it, but I didn't see any of that."

A week after the funeral, Tara's father was admitted to a psychiatric hospital. He would remain there for a year, returning home on weekends and then, progressively, for longer stays. His children's legal guardians were now their maternal uncle and his wife, but they didn't live with them and each night the children would go next door and have supper with their neighbours. Until now, her father had been a lecturer in physiology at King's College. He had a specialty in, and deep fascination with, the human nervous system.

Tara remembers that during his early visits home, her father became manically fixated on the idea of entertaining friends. He would arrange dinner parties and wear his favourite velvet jacket, drink wine and effusively hold court, and then, the next day, return to hospital.

"It frightened me," Tara remembers. "I thought, *How can you be happy?* It was hard trying to navigate grief as a thirteen-year-old and looking to your parental figures to try and have some sense of what it looks like and what's normal or okay. I'm sure he grieved in hospital, but I didn't see it. I had no reference points for grieving. And I probably never realised how much this impacted me until I went to therapy in my thirties."

–

After a year in hospital, their father had returned home. There was no longer the manic enthusiasm, but nor was there an approachable father. Long before her mother's death, Tara had learnt how to tell when her father was depressed, because he would sit in his armchair without a book. He often sat without one now, his vast personal library left untouched.

Within six months of his return, Tara's older sister Jo left home for university. Tara was now fourteen – shy, bereaved and silently craving her sick father's affection. At school she was studious, deferential and painfully self-conscious. She assumed her suffering was a blemish, something socially conspicuous and shameful.

Tara's loneliness and despair didn't present antisocially, and she maintained good grades. But she began smoking and smuggling small quantities of liquor from her oblivious father's cabinet, the booze a social currency she dispensed to friends. She wanted to fit in, to join tribes, and to that end she wore distressed jeans and her dead mother's makeup.

Gravely depressed and emotionally unreceptive, her father was also domestically hapless. Tara would cook for her father, clean and iron his clothes, and explain to him how to use the washing machine and kettle. During this period of caring for her father, she began menstruating and had to clumsily learn the use of tampons by herself. "The ambiguous loss of your father is very hard for people to see or understand," she said. "People understand that when somebody dies, it's clearly traumatic and difficult. They're gone. But the kind of layering of losing Dad, effectively, was not as obvious to others, or even to myself."

—

Grief doesn't always bind the suffering together, nor does it automatically mobilise others' sympathy. Grief is repellent to many – alien, or at least awkward to embrace. And for those sharing the same experience, grief and trauma are formidable pressures that can just as well fracture bonds as intensify them.

After the death of her mother, Tara experienced the loss of both parents. One loss was explicit, the other ambiguous. She expected and desired certain comforts from her father, even if she couldn't at the time describe them, but he retreated alarmingly. For various reasons, Tara's father was incapable of defying his own grief so that he might provide the tender attention and domestic stability so craved by his daughter.

Tara shared a home with her father, and they shared the same loss, but that was all. She felt estranged from him. He was a troubled man but not a callous one, but Tara was perhaps too young to properly acknowledge the distinction.

Tara was obviously pained by her father's "tomb-like" detachment as she grieved her mother, but his detachment also did something else: it left her a lifetime of guilty oscillations between anger and sympathy. She understood the reasons for her father's remoteness, but this knowledge couldn't exorcise her pain. This indeterminacy was exhausting, and one of the legacies of her father's sickness was her guilt about being angry with it.

"I guess I never even thought of my dad as a single father, because I feel like we parented him, really," Tara said. "I really agreed with [English writer J.G.] Ballard when he wrote that the chief threat of a mother's death is an uncaring or absent father. My dad wasn't uncaring, but he was absent, including physically at times when he was in hospital. It's so different to the trauma we experience as firefighters, and there's so much research to show that it's not so much what happens, it's what happens after the event that causes us damage or not."

—

In 1964, J.G. Ballard drove his wife and three children to San Juan, Spain, for a summer holiday. His wife unexpectedly died of pneumonia there, and so, a month later, he made the long drive back to England with his three young, now motherless children. He was thirty-four.

The family of his late wife offered to take custody of the children. Ballard politely declined and became a very rare thing in 1960s Britain: a single father. In dingy, suburban Shepperton, inside days bookended by the ironing of school shirts and the preparation of his children's supper, the widower wrote some of the most imaginative and distinctive prose of the last century. "My greatest ally was the pram in the hall," Ballard wrote in his memoir, *Miracles of Life*, published a year before his death, and referencing Cyril Connolly's famous line: "There is no more sombre enemy of good art than the pram in the hallway."

Only 15 miles away, central London was experiencing historic convulsions of culture, but it was on the city's suburban fringes that Ballard was quietly remaking sci-fi while frying bangers for his kids. "The 1960s were an exciting decade that I watched on television," he wrote at the end of his life.

After he dropped his children at school, Ballard began his working day with a Scotch and soda at 9 a.m. More followed, complemented by a chain of cigarettes. He was, I suppose, a hard-grieving and high-functioning alcoholic, but from the accounts of his children and friends he was also an unusually thoughtful and tender father. And he seemed to be a man who – unlike my grandfather, who lost his wife to brain cancer not long after he returned from Changi's camps, and then vanished for months, leaving his two stunned boys in the care of his siblings – happily revolted against the era's emasculating stigma of single fatherhood.

Like my grandfather, Ballard had been a prisoner of war, captured by the Japanese. But Ballard was a boy during the Second World War, not a soldier, and his experience in Shanghai was much less severe than my grandfather's in Changi. "I have – I won't say happy – not unpleasant memories of the camp," he told a reporter many years later. "I remember a lot of the casual brutality and beatings-up that went on, but at the same time we children were playing a hundred and one games all the time."

The experience was profound, although it took him decades to realise that his novels might all be forms of sublimating it.

He stubbornly resisted suggestions that his florid imagination and recurring metaphors might all derive from his unsettled childhood. I've often wondered if this resistance was the pride of the artist who doesn't want the origins of his imagination made obvious – if he preferred its mystification to its being attributed to "mere" metaphorical reorderings of his childhood. Let me put it another way: I wonder if Ballard ever really thought that his imagination was truly free from his past.

Regardless, his stubbornness lasted until the early 1980s. While writing his enormously successful novel *Empire of the Sun*, published in 1984 and based explicitly upon his time in the camp, he realised that "The memories of Shanghai that I had tried to repress had been knocking at the floorboards under my feet, and had slipped quietly into my fiction."

Those memories included the casual murder of beggars in the street, and, following the Japanese occupancy, his family's sudden transformation from privileged to prisoners. As a boy, the author absorbed a large lesson: seemingly established and imperishable things – family, community, even nations – can be suddenly and violently overturned. "One of the things I took from my wartime experiences was that reality was a stage set," he once told a journalist. "The comfortable day-to-day life, school, the home where one lives and all the rest of it . . . could be dismantled overnight."

His world was upended again in Spain, and for all of Ballard's articulacy, he rarely spoke to his children about their mother's death. He just couldn't do it. Ballard was both an avant-garde writer and a repressed widower. Hundreds or thousands of words were given to his page each day, but his fluency withdrew when his children came home. He could imaginatively interpret modernity, but addressing the grief of his children was beyond him. Instead, his love was expressed with sustained attention and the rituals of domesticity.

And play. In his memoirs, Ballard describes cavorting with his grieving children in the local meadow among detached staircases, severed cars, giant chess pieces and the wooden figurehead of a ship – abandoned props from the local film studio.

It's a lovely triumph: despite the grief, drink and stigma, Ballard still delighted in, and knew the importance of, playing with his children. "Family life has always been important to me, far more important, I suspect, than to people of my parents' generation."

And so, I leave you with another Ballardian image. Not of an empty swimming pool or an abandoned hotel, but of motherless children playing with their grief-sick father in a meadow littered with the old props of cinema. Above them, planes make their low and noisy approach to Heathrow.

—

Unlike Tara's father, Ballard defied his own grief, and others' expectations, by insisting upon his own playfulness with his children. "Dad didn't express his love in rituals of domesticity or sustained attention or play," Tara said. "There was no sustained attention or ability to be present with us. He just wasn't able to do that. Certainly, there wasn't play. Play was not something that I knew. I still struggle to experience play in that kind of carefree, child-like way."

Ballard tried to allow his children to be children. Tara's father couldn't do that, as much as he might have liked. "We became carers for him," she said. "I always, in a way, rescued him. That was what I did, and I took that forward into every relationship, really. That's what I knew. Rescue."

But this wouldn't become obvious for a long time.

—

Tara's parents met at a house party in North London. It was 1966, and Mr Ballard was at home a few kilometres away, writing, drinking and frying bubble and squeak for his children. Bridget was working as a documentary researcher for the BBC, and Shivaji, having completed medical school was now a PhD candidate in physiology. After stealing several glances at the tall blonde across the room, he finally found her eyes and made his way towards her through the crowd.

Tara's father had just finished reading a novel by Bernard Malamud, and his seduction anxiously relied upon discussing it. It worked – or at least it didn't prove repellent – and the two exchanged phone numbers. When picking Bridget up for their first date, Shivaji was quietly gratified to see the book on her mantelpiece. They were married just four months later.

What did they know about each other? Very little. Shivaji knew that his wife's parents weren't pleased about her marrying an Indian man, and he knew she was happily defiant of their bigotry. Bridget knew that her husband was bright and eccentric, but had no understanding yet of his severe depression and bipolar disorder, or of the repressed pains of his childhood.

When Shivaji was six years old, he had left his village of Burhpur for a boat bound for England. It was 1937, and the journey took six weeks. When the ship finally berthed at Tilbury Docks in Essex, Shivaji saw the port's legion of flags and strings of bunting, which were displayed to celebrate the coronation of King George VI, but which he assumed were there to welcome his family to this new country.

Two years later, his new country declared war on Nazi Germany, and not long after that his London neighbourhood was being flattened by the Luftwaffe. For almost sixty consecutive nights, the Germans bombed London, and sometimes they bombed it during the day, too. Children might glimpse a sky suddenly darkened by noisy, death-bearing swarms.

Shivaji's family moved to Basingstoke, about 80 kilometres from the capital, but Hitler's bombers struck there too, including the church they lived beside. By now, Shivaji's father had been called to service as a medical officer with the British Indian Army, leaving Shivaji and his two younger brothers at home with their mother. He would remember his mother fixing a large gas mask to his small face, as clearly as he remembered her admission to a psychiatric ward in 1943.

Young Shivaji didn't then understand schizophrenia, chemical warfare or the ambitions of Hitler – only that he was now parentless. He and his two younger brothers were placed in an orphanage when Shivaji was twelve, and he was unsure what was more frightening: this strange new home, or the weird screams of his mother before she was taken away. Later, a neighbour, Mrs Harding, would foster the three boys.

—

When I was a kid, that's just how he was. Obviously, I didn't understand anything about trauma. It was just Dad, and that's what he did. It was normal for him to block his ears when there was a bottle of champagne being opened, or if there were balloons, he'd go out of the room. Or on firework nights, he'd put headphones on, and he'd just sit there. And you know, we thought that was quite funny – that Dad was scared of fireworks and balloons. Obviously, later on, I sort of had more awareness. But he never spoke about his childhood.

—

Tara was close with her older brother, Adam, and almost reverential of him. In her telling, and from the copious diaries and letters Adam made, he was unusually bright, sensitive and charmingly effusive in his affections.

In 1988, Adam was accepted into Oxford to study chemistry. He was unsure if either the place or the subject suited him, but he squirmed beneath the expectations of his parents. Adam delayed his entrance to Oxford so that he could travel to France and India. In his diary entries and letters home, he sounds like a more mature and affable Holden Caulfield – marked by a hypersensitive dislike for the falsities of society and a torturous uncertainty about how best to deploy his energy and idealism.

Like his father, Adam was a passionate reader, and he confessed to finding a more vibrant and truthful life in the books he read. "Oh God, how I wish that my reality was in the stories I read," he wrote in one diary entry from 1988.

A recurring theme of Adam's diary entries and letters was an intense awareness of his opportunities and a lingering sense that he was incapable of honourably fulfilling them. His letters dazzle with precocious curiosity but are underscored by vicious self-doubt. His obvious intelligence isn't always obvious to him. If he does recognise it, he doesn't seem at all sure that he will find a way to meaningfully express it. They read like the letters and diaries of a bright and sensitive young man still figuring out how to apply his gifts and passions to the world.

Adam was in France on Mother's Day, 1988. He had just finished reading D.H. Lawrence's *Sons and Lovers* and recorded a quote from the novel in his diary, preceded by the words "For me . . .":

> They could not establish between themselves and an outsider just the ordinary human feeling and unexaggerated friendship; they were always restless for something deeper. Ordinary folk seemed shallow to them, trivial and inconsiderable. And so they were unaccustomed, painfully uncouth in the simplest social intercourse, suffering and yet insolent in their superiority. Then beneath was the yearning for soul-intimacy to which

> they could not attain because they were too dumb, and every approach to close connection was blocked by their clumsy contempt of other people. They wanted genuine intimacy, but they could not get even normally near to anyone, because they scorned to take the first steps, they scorned the triviality which forms common human intercourse.

Years later, Tara would see the space between her brother's diaries and his letters. There was a grim uncertainty and self-flagellation in the former. In the letters, Adam would speak of doubt and longing and loneliness, but in a light and apologetic manner designed to partially unburden himself without unduly burdening the recipient.

Much love was expressed between Tara and Adam in letters and postcards. Ardency was hedged by gags, but great feeling was evident despite the cultivated casualness. But privately, in his diaries, Adam's doubt and misery were obvious, and they were clearly more than the ordinary uncertainties of a bright and sensitive young man. After hiking in the Himalayas, he wrote: "Am still feeling that great vacant misery that I left with, and what it is due to, I don't fully understand. All life everywhere in the world suddenly seems small and insignificant, a place where everything is strange and somehow pathetically sad. One could die here and nobody would notice. God, I want some company. I want to see Jo and Ta, and Dad, sweet little Daddy."

His diaries were often like this: within the same paragraph, morbid resignation could suddenly yield to fervent longing.

Fatalism and self-doubt could quickly shift to excitement and the passionate citation of books.

In another entry, made after watching an untouchable caste member scrub the floor of an Indian restaurant on his knees, Adam privately recorded his disgust at the man's debasement – only to then be disgusted by his own vain moralising:

> I wanted to stand up and – in that oh-so-hackneyed way – pull him to his feet and shout to everyone, "This is a man, not a mongrel." Oh fuck it, it's a load of bollocks, but it was the truth. Obligingly, I have written it as it was thought, as tacky and vulgar as it sounded to myself. And, oh how so very patronizing. Great saint gives beggar pride … God, unthinkingly base of me – shit, shut up.

If the diaries captured the painful circularity of his thoughts, they also served as a place to make private affirmations – a place where Adam might reject his previous confessions of depressed inertia. As he was preparing to return to England and take his place at Oxford, he wrote:

> Anyway, I know myself what I should do. I must throw off this doubt and find the courage to make attempts at things, no matter the results. I am not a courageous man, but so long as I am aware of this, then hopefully I shall make myself one. Not a natural courage, but through practice maybe it shall become so. Step forth into the world. I owe so many people, I cannot fail them.

And so, Adam went to Oxford in late 1988 – not triumphantly, but twisted with doubt. Before he did, he left Tara a letter on the kitchen table:

> Dear TJ – Take good care of yourself. I'm going to miss you lots. And baby, even if things look really bad, remember, all of us, Jo, Dad and I, will always be here. If you ever want to talk, just write to me. I will write anyway as no doubt I'm going to feel quite lonely at first as well. All my love, Ad xxx
>
> PS We are all individuals and however incapable we may seem to ourselves we all manage in the end.

As Adam settled into Oxford and Tara remained at home alone with her father, the siblings kept exchanging letters. As he had done from overseas, Adam tried to balance a warm, confiding frankness with a desire not to alarm his sister. He wrote about good grades and boring books; he wrote about his indifference to chemistry and how much he missed his family. He wrote about wanting to change to politics and philosophy, and about the unlikelihood of that happening. He wrote about his love for Tara and acknowledged how hard it must be to live alone with their father.

From university, he wrote:

> However much truth seems weird, it's all we can do to obey it. Heavy concept to stimulate the [older sister] Joji vibes. By the way, send my love to her and to Dad. Maybe he might even

like to write to me? And you, Teej, come up if you want to, we'll go for a piss-up. Until then, little sis, take care and don't let the work get you down. Keep smiling. Love Ad xxx

In October 1988, Adam came down to London for a weekend. He always seemed to have an intuitive sense of others' needs and deployed his charm to accommodate them. But his charm was badly dulled that weekend. His depression mirrored his father's, who was now fixed to his armchair.

Tara was alarmed: something was wrong with her brother. His doubt, modesty and gloomy philosophising no longer seemed like mere parts of a restlessly bright mind.

Now, they seemed like fixtures. Adam was genuinely tortured – the pain was real, not poetically exaggerated.

–

Tara sat for her own Oxford entrance exam that year. She did so nervously, and with the expectation that she'd fail. She wasn't much interested in going there, and never expected to, but she was satisfying her father's desire that she try. There was one exam question she remembers: *Can someone else be a better judge of my interests than I am myself?*

It was a stunningly open question, enticing for some but intimidating for others, and Tara stumbled on it. She recognised that the question was there to prompt the pen of the most brilliantly discursive, but she could only think of her brother, and her response recorded her anxiety about his health.

As Tara had taught her father how to work a kettle and taught herself how to insert a tampon, she was now also becoming gravely worried about her brother but unsure how to help him.

On 21 November 1988, Adam wrote the following in his diary:

> I want to write a final statement of what I am. I am weak-willed, lazy, insecure and very stupid. I wasn't once, that's true. However, I have been living by that fact for a number of years now. Everybody believes it isn't true, but unfortunately it is. All life is passing me by now. The only way I see it in some part of its fire is unfortunately when I am drunk, when not worried by anything in the world. The rest of the time it is a chore, a dream waiting to end. The only reason for this is because I have made it so, by convincing myself that this is what it is like. But these words do actually have meaning. Unfortunately I also realize that I cannot live like this because there are so many people that love me in all honesty. I cannot match their love and so I cannot allow myself to destroy them as I have destroyed myself. My whole life has been a catharsis – look at my "writings".

This wasn't precocious fretfulness but terminal self-loathing.

—

Tara was woken by the phone. It was just after two in the morning of 22 November 1988. Alone in bed, she wondered who would be calling in the middle of the night. Then she heard her father climb the stairs and knock on her bedroom door. "It's Adam," he said. "He's had an accident. He's in hospital. I have to go to Oxford."

There was no more information, and Tara asked if she could go with him. Her father said no, that she should stay there, and so she did – lying in bed, sick with anxiety and a sense of helplessness. She watched the digital clock beside her bed, anticipating the ringing of the phone. She was scared, nauseous and resentful that she couldn't go with her father.

There was no sleep, of course, and without company those hours were long and sharp. The phone rang again around 6.30 a.m. It was a neighbour, telling her that Adam was in hospital – something she already knew. There was no more detail, no new information that might alleviate her fear. But there was one thing: Tara's second Oxford entrance exam was that morning, and her neighbour passed on her father's desire that she sit for it.

She didn't, but she still went to school. Then she waited for her sister Jo to come and drive them both to the Oxford hospital where Adam lay. She felt powerless. Overwhelmingly powerless.

—

The previous evening, Adam had left a final note on his desk beside a pack of Marlboro cigarettes and jumped from the high window of his dorm room. He was found unconscious and gravely injured and taken to the local hospital. He lay there unresponsive for nine days, his life artificially sustained by machines, while his eyes remained partially opened – promising his family their full disclosure. But the damage was mortal, and the machines were eventually turned off.

Tara would later write: "Why would you choose to terminate that hope? Switching off the life support feels like driving a suicide bomb into your family home. I wanted to cling to my brother's beating heart, and so did my father."

Tara didn't receive any sedatives, but there's a good reason why they should have been offered. The pain is incomprehensible, and you can only wish for the impossible: for the reversal of time; for the replacement of your own skin. In this hell, sleep is one of your few friends. And time. So much time.

—

It was Christmas Eve, 1988, and just a month had passed since Adam's death. Depressed by the sight of her unresponsive father, that evening Tara vainly sought escape from her grief and domestic claustrophobia – and to pretend, if only for a few hours, that she "was a normal teenage girl".

She arranged with friends to meet at a pub – the Wells Tavern in Hampstead, a place where Adam used to drink – and so they did, but the drunk merriment was painfully incongruous and Tara ran away towards Hampstead Heath. Her friend Dan followed.

And so they walked the hills together and saw the lights of London below, and then they walked some more, off the paths now and into the high grass and trees, and then Tara stopped and fell to her knees and screamed and wept while down below, somewhere among the city's lights, her father sat at home in his armchair.

—

Tara wasn't yet twenty when Adam died, but she now feared her own death and the deaths of others with a special intensity. She was also moved by something else. Tara wanted a rich and purposeful vocation, something that would honour her brother. She wanted her labour to observably touch the world.

There was a parlous stacking of expectations here: the expectation that Tara live a life that was worthy of her brother, who in turn had borne the expectations of their dead mother. Here was a young woman trying to honour the will of ghosts, forging her future via correspondence with the dead. In 1990, Tara went to Edinburgh University to study physiology. There were the usual privations of student life – an unvarying diet of beans and toast, eaten in a room without heating, her breath visible in the winter. From her bedroom window, she could see Arthur's Seat, the extinct volcano and the city's solemn fixture. She loved all of it – everything except the work itself.

Tara drank, smoked and made new friends. She went swimming and learnt to windsurf. She barely studied. Bored by her subject and excited to find that her grief had eased enough to allow a social life and flashes of happiness, she enjoyed every other part of college life.

Then, one day, Tara learnt of a campus computer that would take certain personal details, process them via inscrutable algorithms and, after mysterious consideration, suggest your ideal career. She submitted her information, and the prophet made two suggestions: physiotherapist or firefighter. In turn, she would become both. "I think that computer absolutely changed the course of my life," Tara said. "Because I don't think that seed would have ever been there otherwise. I never would have even thought about it. [Firefighting] was something that was so far out of the realm of anything I'd ever considered."

But it wasn't the only influence. "When I reflect on it now, and in my research and speaking with lots of firefighters, you see how many people in emergency services have a history of trauma," she said. "And so: was that the best career for me? I don't know. But when I experienced those losses at a young age, it threatened my whole sense of safety in the world. I didn't think the world was safe. [I thought] that anything could happen and that people could die at any time – and they *did* die. And so I wanted things to be black and white, right and wrong, which is quite a normal response to trauma."

–

In 1995, when she was twenty-four, Tara fell in love with Australia and then with Anthony. She was enchanted by Sydney, by its prettiness for a city so large, its beaches and sunshine. These are the clichéd virtues of the place, but they're real, and Tara felt them deeply. So had her mother, years before Tara was born, when she visited in the early 1960s; she later named one of her daughter's teddy bears "Sydney".

"Part of it was being free from the expectations of me that I felt back in the UK, from all the history and the memories," Tara said. "But it was more than that. It was also about the outdoor lifestyle. It's really easy to be happy here for me, to be able to live near the ocean and to be outside in the sunlight. If I can go outside and get to the beach every day and get on the water, or in it, or just look at it, then that's such a simple pleasure that's just there. I know there's so many great aspects of London, but they're not the things that really bring me alive, and most of that is the outdoors – the ocean and the mountains."

Tara came on a working holiday visa, and waited tables at a nightclub near Circular Quay. That's where she met Anthony, a handsome bloke who impressed Tara with his ocker serenity.

Tara adored him immediately but, assuming she was unworthy and pre-empting heartbreak, she disguised her adoration and talked up the value of friendship versus romance. She interpreted Anthony's kindnesses to her as merely democratic, while he interpreted her coyness as romantic indifference. In this way, months passed before their mutual attraction was realised.

They both lived in Bondi, and they first kissed on its beach, and from then they were inseparable. They worked together, swam together, went rock-climbing together. Seeing Tara at her apartment window one day from the street, he scaled the building with a rose between his teeth. "It was young love," Tara would write many years later. "Young, innocent, lustful, uncomplicated love."

Perhaps for a while, but their love would become complicated – first by the pending expiration of her visa, and then by the rising pitch of emotional dissonance that Tara had, for a time, so successfully ignored.

–

Tara's visa expired, and after leaving Australia she flew to New Zealand, where she tried to purge her heartache and internal quivering with sky-diving and white-water rafting. She wrote letters to Anthony and went hiking through mountain ranges, and felt guilty that she couldn't properly admire, or be at peace with, the natural beauty. Tara wanted what her brother had sought and Wordsworth had found: "to connect the landscape with the quiet of the sky". But her mind was too busy, and one night in her tent she experienced what she would only recognise years later as a panic attack.

Six weeks later, she returned to gloomy London and worked as a waitress in a café. The gloom was brightened by news that Anthony would soon visit her – and then brightened some more when he arrived and suggested she move to Australia, apply for residency and move in with him.

Tara was ecstatic. Had he asked her to marry him, she's certain she would have said yes. Her father gave his blessing to the move, and Tara moved permanently to Australia in 1996.

But they were young, and Anthony's love was more fickle than either of them realised. Within a year or two, he confessed that he no longer loved her and admitted a mutual attraction to a friend of hers. They attended one session of couple's therapy together, where Tara received her first sense that her childhood was influencing her behaviour in relationships. Desirous of love but fearful of pain, she could undermine them by anticipating their dissolution.

"It was whilst working as a physiotherapist in my early thirties, and triggered by the ending of another dysfunctional relationship, that I began my own personal journey of healing," Tara would write in the introduction to her doctoral thesis many years later. "A convoluted path that would weave its way through the next two decades of my life as I tried to make sense of myself and my story. With the support of a psychologist, and later a psychotherapist, I revisited my childhood, peeling back the layers of myself that I had created in an unconscious attempt to keep myself safe. It was effortful, painful, and challenging."

It took time to become conscious of long-unconscious behaviour. Of how she gravitated towards men she felt might need saving, and kept her own vulnerability hidden. How she felt that no man, once he'd seen all her psychic scars, could ever really love her.

Between her own heart and her partner's, Tara had unconsciously imposed an elaborate and impossible maze. She wanted to keep herself safe, and she also wanted love, and these two desires were tragically incompatible. Today, Tara said, she attributes the fact that she never married or had kids to her childhood and the fears it created – fears that were normalised so early that for a long time, she rarely acknowledged them.

When Tara talked about her difficulty in relationships, and the fact that she had never married or had children, I thought of her mother's letter and its aspiration that she would find fulfillment in both. "For a long time, I really felt that sense of failure," Tara said. "And it was really a sense of failure that I had let her down. I think that probably, on a subconscious level, my own sense of failure for not having children was strengthened because of what she'd written in the letter. But some of [that sense of failure] was my own.

"But that's changed, and I have done work on allowing myself to feel angry with my mum, maybe not specifically around the letter that she wrote to me, but certainly around the letter she wrote to my brother, and what that meant to him.

"I guess the relationship I have with my mum now is very different. I know that she would be proud of me, that she loved me, and she would still love me. I know that, and that's enough now. And I can see the fraughtness of her trying to write, knowing she was dying, and trying to express so much in just one little letter."

—

The request came from police, and it was a simple but macabre job. It was September 2009, and a man had just killed himself by jumping from an apartment window in Darlinghurst. Police had removed his body from the pavement, but much blood was left behind, and they'd asked the firies to wash it away with their hoses.

Also left on the pavement were the dead man's shattered glasses, which Tara picked up before she began washing the footpath clean. As she watched the blood and water disappear down the drain, she thought idly that she was washing away some final essence of the stranger.

And then she thought of Adam. She looked up towards the window the stranger had leapt from and thought of her brother leaping from his. She wondered whether there was a moment between his jumping and landing when he experienced the briefest but most acute regret. She looked back to the footpath and felt a tightening in her chest as she watched the last of the blood vanish down the street's grate.

Her colleague that day knew nothing of Tara's past – few of them did. Back in the fire truck, he wondered incredulously about suicide. It seemed so baffling, he said. *Who would do that?*

Tara felt nauseous. She stayed silent. Tried regulating her breathing; tried quelling the nausea as her colleague riffed obliviously.

She thought about how her uniform had imposed a firewall upon her psyche. Her vulnerability, insecurity and avoidance existed only in civilian clothes. When she was wearing the uniform, she could fulfill its expectations and exist proudly as a resilient, competent and socially useful human being.

It was, of course, the same psyche – but the delineation was useful to her. Now, she saw her civilian past graphically collide with her role as firefighter. She had washed the blood of a stranger from a footpath, just as someone must've washed her brother's blood from an Oxford courtyard. The uniform could help her to compartmentalise – it could help her to avoid certain truths – but it was not impervious. Now, she experienced the collapse of the firewall and became, simultaneously, a firefighter and grief-plagued sister. She had always hoped to keep the two identities separate, until, perhaps, one grew strong enough to nullify the other.

Back at the station, the boys were surprisingly tender. They didn't know Tara's history, but they could see she was upset. One brought chocolates and tissues to her room. Touched, Tara told the young firefighter the story of Adam's death. She hadn't meant to, but she was glad she did.

The culture of emergency services can be unforgiving, often necessarily. Colleagues depend upon each other with a particular intensity, and this requires mutual faith in one another's competence and stability. To confess sadness or trauma might be interpreted as weakness and undermine trust. Many emergency workers will conceal trouble lest it encourage collegial suspicion. In some cases, emotional distress – whether wrought by work or carried from the past – may well render a person unreliable.

On the other hand, a colleague's past, once shared, may strengthen bonds. Tara found this to be true after the Darlinghurst suicide. She had acquitted a simple job, but one that colleagues now saw had been uniquely harrowing for her, and they responded compassionately.

There's no formula for when a personal confession might strengthen the fraternity. Emergency workers are, typically, literal and goal-focused individuals and wary of undue philosophising or personal disclosure. But they are not automatons, and personal disclosure can deepen sympathy and loyalty if those disclosures are made by competent colleagues (perceived competency will often determine how receptive colleagues are). After Tara told her colleagues about Adam, she realised the benefit of not pretending that she was preternaturally resilient. And she felt some relief.

The Darlinghurst suicide happened only a few days before Adam's birthday. He would have been forty-one. On that day, 16 September, Tara walked down to the beach. She sat on the sand and looked out over the ocean. She experienced no revelation, had no fresh insights into her brother's death or her own life. She just felt a heavy, imponderable sadness.

When she got home, she wrote a letter to Adam. The writing was raw, unconsidered. It just came out, and she had no interest in polishing it.

> Dear Adam,
>
> Today you should have been turning forty-one. How I would have loved to share this day with you, to drink a glass of wine and make a toast together, to have a run together or a game of tennis or even just to annoy each other as we always used to. Remember that game we played where we would climb on each other's shoulders and one of us would hang from the cornice in the living room while the other would see how many times they could run back and forth before they had to pick the other up? Or remember the time you kicked that door and then had to limp around for weeks after?

You always protected me, you looked after me – I loved that. I am as sad now as I was twenty-one years ago when you died. The sadness never leaves. I can only carry those memories with me and imagine the person you would have been today. Would you have been married? Would you have kids? What would you be doing and where would you be living? I know you would have led an amazing life, a caring life. You would have made a difference to people's lives. Even now, even without life, you still do. I wish you knew that. Only yesterday I received an email from an old school friend whom I haven't seen in many years wanting to include you as part of a living tribute art project in Trafalgar Square. I declined; I didn't think you would want that. Was I right? Would you have wanted to be remembered publicly in Trafalgar Square? I think not, but perhaps it was my own selfishness that said no. To me you are mine. What we shared is ours. You are not a statistic, you are my brother, and I alone understand why you did what you did, or at least that's how it feels, and that is what I cling to – that intimacy and closeness to you. Something that is so starkly clear that I lack in my life, something that I yearn for. I guess I protect you in your death as fiercely and tenderly as you protected me in your life. Cheers to you, my gorgeous brother, on your forty-first birthday. I love you now as I always did. Your big little sister x

Tara can still feel embarrassment or even shame when discussing the Darlinghurst suicide, so slight does it seem in comparison to some of her colleagues' experiences on the job.

She understands why it had such an impact on her, but said: "When I read other people's stories … [I] go, 'Oh my God, you've experienced horrendous scenes.' And so, there's a certain amount of shame attached to me – that was a very simple job, you know. And most of my trauma was prior to entering the job."

–

After several years posted to various metropolitan fire stations, Tara was tiring. She came to anxiously anticipate the station's bells, and in 2016 she sought to replace them with the ring of telephones: she applied for a transfer to the emergency dispatch centre. Her induction, via an intense training course, was very different from Peter James's in the 1970s, when the sum of his training for emergency dispatch was an encouraging pat on the back.

Two call centres served the state of New South Wales, one in Sydney and the other in Newcastle, and both were staffed by serving firefighters. On Tara's Sydney desk sat four computer screens, where calls were listed, their details logged, and maps of the caller's location displayed. She answered triple zero calls from the public, calls from other government bodies such as the Environment Protection Authority, monitored radio comms and dispatched trucks.

The public's calls were the most stressful. A dispatcher may have to advise a stranger in life-threatening conditions, often with imperfect knowledge and limited resources to deploy.

The dispatcher needs to solicit as much information as they can from the caller, but the caller's panic or confusion can make this difficult. Sometimes they might simply scream or plead. "You're giving people information about, say, should they stay in their house? Or should they leave their house? And if I make the wrong decision, and tell them to stay? It depends on the situation: have they got enough time to leave? Have they adequately prepared their house for bushfire? Do they have any static water supply? Should they stay, or should they go? And if you make the wrong decision ..."

The dispatcher must triage jobs, as well as classify them – will a specialist HAZMAT crew be required, or structural engineers? The dispatcher will want to know if people are trapped, if toxic chemicals are present, and what type of building is threatened, so that the right crew can be deployed with the appropriate degree of urgency. "There is an automated dispatch system," Tara said. "But it depends upon what information you put into [it]."

Determining the precise location of the emergency is more easily done for metro jobs than for rural ones. When Tara took a call, typically from a mobile phone, a map of the caller would appear on one of her screens. The precision of this was much greater in the city, where mobile towers are vastly more abundant. For certain rural calls, an unhelpfully large radius – sometimes as great as 50 kilometres – could circle the caller. If the caller was away from home and did not have a specific address or major landmark to refer to, the dispatcher would have to rely upon the caller's descriptions. If the caller found themselves trapped on a country road with fire bearing down upon them, they may only have a small hill and some undistinguished trees to offer as guides.

"That can be quite stressful," Tara said. "All they want to know is that somebody's coming, and they're screaming, and you're trying – you know you've got to get something on the road – but in order to do that, you've got to locate them, and that isn't always easy."

During a major bushfire, the number of available trucks is limited, and the call centre would often be overwhelmed by calls, many from people not directly threatened by the fire but who were anxious to report their sighting of smoke. For one incident, countless witnesses might call triple zero; Tara would watch the calls piling up on her screen, certain that most would relate to the same fire, but with no way of knowing which involved a mortal threat, and which might relate to an entirely different emergency.

This context of high stakes, limited resources and imperfect information increases the chances of anguish – of either making a decision that results in catastrophe, or of simply feeling shamefully inadequate in the face of profound need. "There were a couple of colleagues that were always just very, very calm – *really* calm – and were able to ask the right questions and multitask and were able to accurately use the system to pinpoint where somebody was very, very quickly," Tara said. "This absolute calmness, not allowing the energy of whoever's on the end of the phone to be taken onboard – I don't think that I was fantastic at that. I think I did get stressed. I wasn't the worst person there at all, but I wasn't the best, either. And I think my own lack of confidence played on me, you know, and I was always thinking that I'd done something wrong."

There was also always the possibility of hearing, on the other end of the line, supreme terror – nightmare sounds compounded by the dispatcher's relative helplessness. Sometimes those sounds would stop abruptly, followed by the silence of death.

Tara expresses relief that she never took such a call, but she worked with plenty who did. "I had colleagues who were trying to help somebody trapped in a house fire with how to exit, and hearing them screaming, and the line going dead, and [they] have subsequently experienced PTSD from those sorts of jobs."

In 2009, Jeannie Van Den Boogaard was working as a dispatcher for the Victorian Emergency Services Telecommunications Authority. On the day of the Black Saturday bushfires, 7 February, when some 400 separate fires were recorded in Victoria, she was rostered for a twelve-hour shift. Via high winds and historic heat, many fires conjoined and became fire storms. They were the most fatal bushfires in Australia's history: 187 people died. Thousands of homes were destroyed; whole towns were almost extinguished. Of Marysville, population 500, the Victorian premier said on 11 February: "There's no activity, there's no people, there's no buildings, there's no birds, there's no animals, everything's just gone."

Van Den Boogaard started her shift in the early afternoon, assuming responsibility for the radio dispatch of the Community Fire Authority's Region 13. "Not long after I slipped my headset on, the fires took off through the Kinglake region, and within about twenty minutes I was dealing with a horrific mayday call from a crew whose fire truck had become disabled, and they had the fire bearing down on them," she told a 2018 federal senate inquiry. "That was only the start of my shift."

Van Den Boogaard, in both her written submissions and oral testimony, described the "madness and mayhem" in the control centre and the "anguish" of those on the frontline. "Most people think of Black Saturday as a one-day event, when, in actual fact, it went on for weeks," she said. "I, like others, went back in, shift after shift, even on my days off during those weeks. Unfortunately, as a result, I now have PTSD, severe depression and anxiety. I went to work one day, and I came home a different person whose life has been changed forever."

But Van Den Boogaard didn't know she had PTSD. Not then, and not for a long time after. She knew that she'd changed – that she was sadder, more anxious. But she continued in the job until, almost exactly five years after 7 February 2009, she received a call from a stricken woman reporting an approaching fire. "It's just like Black Saturday all over again," the woman said.

Those words vibrated terribly with Van Den Boogaard. They were "the straw that broke the camel's back", she told the inquiry, and when she heard them, she wept at her desk. A colleague shepherded her to the staff kitchen, where she sat numbly and realised, at last, that she was sick and could do this no longer.

A strange and torturous part of the job, especially for those with operational experience, is that it both acutely adrenalises you *and* chains you to a desk. The sympathetic nervous system is constantly provoked, but the mental circuit of signal/response is never completed. The dispatcher, uncertain of their influence or of the outcome of the job, simply moves to the next call.

"You often don't have a sense of agency," Tara said. "You can't do anything. Your heart rate's going, but you're just on the end of the phone. At least when you're [on the frontline], you're physically working and releasing all of that stress response, and you've got some agency over what happens. Whereas when you're sitting in the call centre, you're just sitting still."

It's a vital job, but for certain men and women, a sense of helplessness is a curse. After three years in dispatch, Tara was again craving operational duty. She felt the encroachment of burnout again; she was now anticipating calls as anxiously as she had once anticipated the station's bells. It was time to return to the station.

—

In 2018, while still an operational firefighter, Tara began a PhD with the University of New England. Informed by her experience as a member of Fire and Rescue NSW's critical incident and peer support team, her doctoral thesis was titled *A Violation of Coherence: A Narrative Inquiry Study of Firefighters' Experiences of Exposure to Suicide*. In its introduction, she explained her motivation for writing it. "In my role as a peer, and through working with firefighters for many years, I repeatedly heard their stories of trauma and suicide," she wrote. "I saw their distress and pain, how it both mirrored and differed from my own. The challenges they faced with understanding and making sense of suicide were, at times, palpable, and they would turn to me for answers. During this time, I was myself exposed to suicide occupationally as a firefighter, and I experienced a visceral reaction that unravelled further layers of trauma. These occupational experiences not only led me to want to conduct this research but also significantly influenced the derivation of the research question."

By now, Tara's old fear of uncertainty and ambiguity had mellowed. Her perspective had shifted, she wrote, "from science, positivism, and a desire (verging on a need) for absolute truth towards an intuitive 'sniffing out' of narrative qualitative research, finding joy rather than fear, in the inherent 'messiness' and ambiguity of it".

For Tara's research, she interviewed twenty firefighters, most of them still active. Each had encountered suicide, either professionally or personally, and in most cases both: several had lost multiple friends, colleagues or family members to suicide and had attended many scenes of self-annihilation.

Tara had thought of herself as an attentive listener, but listening back to the interviews, she realised she wasn't as good as she thought she was. For one, their stories' resonance with her own could distract her, as she found herself experiencing surges of memory or empathy. She also had to temper her instinct to silently project her own experience onto theirs, and she had to get better at absorbing awkward silences – at sitting patiently with another's pauses, however lengthy. "It really taught me to allow people to have space in the silence to contemplate and ruminate on what they wanted to say," she said. "I heard myself jump in a few times and was a bit horrified ... that was a really important learning experience for me. I had a lot to learn about deep listening."

Their responses weren't uniform, but there were distinct patterns. Emotion, for many, was something to be feared, as both a sign of weakness and a threat to their own professionalism. Most saw themselves as "rescuers and protectors", Tara thought, and their social, professional and inner lives were governed by this belief, just as hers had been. Granite resilience was necessary not only for their job, but also for their self-conception, and encounters with suicide threatened this on several fronts. They couldn't help prevent it; they couldn't comprehend the dead's motivation for killing themselves, and their subsequent emotion threatened their sense of resilience, which was valorised both personally and by the culture around them.

Tara repeatedly saw how her participants' incomprehension of suicide had shaken their assumptions about the world. They were disoriented. Many also felt guilty. They were protectors, but if they couldn't ultimately protect their best friends, they wondered how useful they really were. To these unstable compounds of incomprehension, grief and guilt were added the sparks of anger and a complicated sense of betrayal.

Some respondents, electrified by anxiety, were conversationally scattered. Others assumed a stoic pose, even as they choked upon their recollections. One feared for his teenage child, who had recently been diagnosed with depression. Another expressed bafflement at his own emotional numbness. One firefighter couldn't purge the recurring image of a body. "I found it hard to be at the station ... particularly when it came to going to sleep, I kept thinking I would see him. It was weird ... I still remember it pretty vividly. I still know it's there. I can think about it and be there."

Her participants displayed avoidance and detachment. Some of this seemed healthy and proportionate; other examples suggested a terrible emotional alienation. Several of her subjects' marriages had broken down.

After each interview, Tara recorded how the conversations had affected her. "There were many things that Tony said that resonated with my own story, yet it didn't trigger me, perhaps because it was not overtly emotional and there were no tears," she wrote in her journal. "There was a real sense of 'Pandora's box', a mountain of repressed emotion, a story untold."

–

Late 2024 was a bitterly disorienting time for Tara. While her PhD had been approved that year, she saw a trilogy of endings: of her father's life, her physical health and her firefighting career. She was forced to choose that last ending – her injuries now precluded operational work, but she was offered other, desk-bound, roles – and it now mixed with the others, and the freedom of pursuing new things invited more fear than excitement.

After almost twenty years in the service, Tara had grown tired, jaded. She had once submitted happily to its regimented structure, but now, as her need for structure and stability mellowed, found it less hospitable. Twenty years ago, she had found a second family and great purpose in the job. Neither of those things had been nullified, but she felt emptied now. Then, she had seen all the possible ways she might be helpful. Now, she thought more about how bureaucratic systems might thwart those attempts to help. She retired in November 2024.

Her physical health didn't help. In recent years, she'd badly torn her hamstring, had it surgically reattached, then experienced post-surgery infection. In late 2024 she required hip surgery. It wasn't the pain of the injuries that distressed Tara, but how they might affect her athleticism – so much of her pleasure, her sense of vitality and connection with the world, came from great hikes and physical exploration.

After her surgery, as she lay in her hospital bed, she received a call from her sister in London. Their father had died. The next day, as nurses helped Tara from her bed, she collapsed. "I don't know what happened," she said. "But I was gone for some time. I could hear the voices of people standing, worried, around me. There was a young physio there, and I think it scared her. It sounds very dramatic, but I thought I was dying, because I could hear voices but I couldn't respond in any way."

She had returned to England several times in her father's last years. She knew the end was close and had painfully speculated as to when it might come, so that she could be there with him. She wanted to hold her father's hand as he died, as he'd requested. "He said, 'The one thing I want is for both of my daughters to be holding my hand when I die,'" Tara said, weeping. "And I tried so hard. I went there last year and sat for seven weeks next to him, and he was like, 'Why won't they let me die?' And then he died the one day when I couldn't be there. He'd been dying for eighteen months, and I'd been there for five weeks in June, and then he died the one day that I was completely helpless in hospital . . . I know it's going to take me a while to process what that really means for me."

Her grief blended with anger and guilt – a familiar mixture. Tara confronted not only the loss of her second parent, but all the other grievances that come with grief. She felt angry with her father and then guilty about her anger.

–

How do you write a eulogy, and who is it for? Is it for the dead, for the speaker or for the mourners? A eulogy can subtly writhe with conflict. If the writer is eulogising her father on behalf of her siblings, can they agree upon who he was? Even if they can, do they agree about what to emphasise?

Tara appreciated her sister's faith in her and the freedom to write the eulogy independently, but she faced a problem: how to balance authenticity with respect? She wanted to be honest about his life of great suffering, without disrespecting the dead or alienating the living by being excessively morbid. Her eulogy would have to thread the eye of a needle.

But how? How to soulfully and respectfully render a man whose life was so insistently marked by despair? A man who once told Tara that he would have long ago slit his throat were it not for his daughters. A man who studied the human nervous system while his own was still trembling from Nazi bombs. A man who lost his wife to cancer and his son to suicide and almost lost his two daughters to his deep, grief-made retreat. A man who, after losing his wife, gave his money away, spurned his friends and thought Russian spies were following him. A man who often spoke of welcoming his own death.

How do you eulogise such a life? And who is the eulogy for? I asked Tara about this, before she had written the eulogy and before she left for London. "I find it really hard," she said, "because, he's not somebody that, once he got to the end of a long life, you think: 'Let's look back and reflect upon this wonderful long life he had.' I really have struggled with that – how to be authentic and real without it just being really depressing."

–

A week after her farewell from the fire brigade, in November 2024, Tara flew to London for her father's funeral. On the long flight, she willed herself to write the eulogy, but once she landed in London, she still felt incapable of raising a pen or opening a laptop.

She met with an old friend who had known Adam, and Tara asked her a favour. Could she dictate the speech to her? Her friend agreed and became Tara's patient stenographer. They completed the eulogy together. In a chapel, Tara assumed the lectern before her father's coffin:

"Our dad was one of life's great mysteries, a unique wonder of the world. When letting my friends know of his death, I said my gentle, tortured dad has died – and he was gentle and tortured, but he was also charismatic and passionate with a brilliant mind that burst with ideas, and he could be very, very funny. In many ways he was a living paradox …

"We loved to see him laugh, especially as for so much of his life he was so sad. Dad struggled with mental illness throughout his life, beginning during his childhood. He rarely spoke of the trauma of that time, except to say that he had no doubt he had many repressed memories. And he experienced several hospital admissions whilst we were growing up.

"Then our mum, Bridget, battled cancer for five years before she died in May 1984, when I was thirteen, Adam was fifteen and Jo was seventeen, devastating our family. Dad struggled to cope with the loss, and for a while he was admitted again to a psychiatric hospital. It was during this time that we received so much love, kindness and support from so many people who are here today. You saved us in the way that Mrs Harding saved our dad and his brothers. And we want to say a heartfelt thank you, not only from us, but also from our dad.

"As you all know, the pain of our childhood weighed heavily on our beloved brother, Ad. And on 21 November 1988 – thirty-six years ago next week – when he was in his first term at Oxford University, he took his own life. For Dad, this was simply too much to bear. He retreated from life to live quietly with his books in Norfolk …

"I want to leave you with this image of Dad, sunken deep into his favourite brown armchair in our living room, surrounded by his book collection, captivated by the story he is reading, nodding, smiling, chuckling to himself, oblivious to the world around him – happy and at peace."

And then a series of photos played on the chapel's TV screens. Photos of a smiling young man; then photos of a smiling young father; then photos of a smiling older father – without context, they might seem to testify to a happy, unblighted life, surrounded by love and books and happy adventures. Ella Fitzgerald's "Isn't It Romantic?" played with the carousel of pictures.

During the service, the priest stressed that for as long as people remembered Shivaji, he would never truly be dead – independent of heaven, those on Earth could spiritually sustain his life through their memories. These were standard lines of comfort at a funeral, and I don't mean to even faintly mock them. But Tara wondered about the meaning of a life that her father was often indifferent to keeping. Her memories of her father inspired anger as much as gratitude, pity as much as awe. She needed no encouragement to keep her father's memory alive, but the idea that those memories would automatically provide comfort was less assured.

"I did a lot of work trying to heal my relationship with my dad and accept him for what he was and what he was able to give me," Tara told me after the funeral. "And accepting that he was never going to be the dad I wanted him to be. And I think that was a huge part of [healing our relationship]. I mean, we were never going to have the relationship that I wanted and hoped for and kind of desperately craved, really, especially after Mum died. But it was definitely better.

"As we get older, the situations change, but I think there were many aspects of that relationship that remained a bit lopsided in a way, because we became carers for him ... He was, in a way, very much the child – the broken child – and a victim, and I always needed to make sure he was okay somehow. But then that didn't leave enough space for me to be okay. Do you know what I mean? And so [a major job for me was] trying to hold that and be able to love him but be angry with him at the same time. And that's something I still find really difficult – how to love people but still be allowed to be angry with them for being let down by them."

—

When I spoke with Tara's sister Jo, I asked about her mother's letters to her three children – the shadow of them, and Tara's long and painful interpretation of hers. Jo considered them very differently in one crucial, simple way: that the letters were written in order of the children's birth, and their coherence, attention and care diminished as their mother progressively got sicker. In other words, the differences between the letters mostly reflected their writer's diminishing health. "Regarding the quality of the letters themselves – she got sicker and sicker and sicker, and I think she must have done it in chronological order, because mine was perfect. I mean, perfectly formed. [Whereas] I don't know if my sister's was [even] signed or finished.

"The intention was to leave a message to her children. But I think they were unfortunate in the sense that I think it put a lot of burden on my brother to achieve things that maybe ... Well, it was a big burden for him. And I think the fact that Tara's was unfinished would have put a burden on her."

There's sorrow here. Sorrow in the failure of the sisters to compare notes, which might perhaps have allowed Tara to find some comfort in her sister's theory. And sorrow in contemplating that Tara's lifetime of faint anguish might have been caused by nothing more than accident or tragic happenstance: that her mother's love and ambition for her was no less than she held for her other children, but that simply, because Tara was the youngest child, her mother's final statement to her was the one most weakened by her terminal illness.

—

Brett Kersten embraced the paramilitary structure of the police force – or perhaps it's more accurate to say that he was grateful that it embraced him. He never really lost his faith in authority, nor in the comfort that followed his absorption into its formal structures.

Tara was similar, in a way. The tragedies and rolling disorder of her childhood left her craving both control and a proxy family. Firefighting offered the bonds of kinship; it seemed a worthy life, and one that her late brother would have approved of. But her contentment with her work, and her very engagement with the world, changed over time. When we spoke a few days after the farewell ceremony marking the end of her almost twenty years of service, she said that there were two halves to her career: the first half was exciting and fulfilling; the second was marked by frustration, exhaustion and a sense that the organisational rigidity had left her "fighting to be valued, heard, seen".

"Before you even say your name, you say your number – your service number," Tara said. "I think all of that is damaging to being a human. And I've always found it incredibly difficult to have any sort of meaningful conversation with anybody who was of a higher rank than me, when you're standing in uniform and you have to call them 'Sir'."

Emergency response demands discipline and submission to the organisational whole, so perhaps it can't be any other way. But Tara herself changed over the years of her firefighting career. She craved control less, and she came to accept and even rejoice in her individualism. The comforts of fraternity became less important than her own fulfillment and expression. In the second half of her career, Tara was more likely to grate against petty officiousness and her feeling of anonymity than to feel gratitude for a sense of belonging. "It was death by a thousand cuts," she said. "My disillusionment really had more to do with organisational stuff, rather than trauma exposure."

I sensed from Tara, as she reflected on her career in the days following her retirement, a faint but bitterly held belief that some unspoken accord had not been upheld – that she had given a very large and important part of herself to the job but had not received commensurate care in return.

"I felt so angry and resentful about my career for a long time," she said. "I didn't want to feel that way, and I kind of worked through that to a point ... by the time I left, I stopped feeling so angry and it was kind of nice to be able to make peace with it."

The dramatic convergence of events following her retirement – the tide of tender reflection after her farewell; her surgery and uncertain health; the death of her father – meant her retirement felt scary and her future uncertain. After a few months, her fear had mellowed. She now saw the blankness of her future not as an abyss but as a clear canvas. This reflected a fundamental emotional and philosophical change – one that, I suspect, made her no longer an ideal candidate for emergency services, with its command-and-control structure and well-defined roles. Tara no longer worshipped control in the abstract. She could now see its semi-illusory nature and all the sacrifices she'd made in attempting to secure it. She could now, as she told me, sit with the irresolution of things. "I had shifted through time and really through my own healing process, from being quite sword-like and black and white and not wanting any uncertainty to being able to sit in the messiness of it all. Through a lot of therapy, I changed my whole world view and belief systems – from not really wanting to embrace the fact that life was chaos, essentially, and everything was full of uncertainty, to kind of knowing that it was and it is and embracing that. In fact, that's where magic can happen."

As a child, Tara imagined her own complicity in the death and disorder that afflicted her family. Years later, if she's still a guilt-stricken and compulsive apologiser, that quality is, happily, much softened.

I thought of the question Tara faced in her first Oxford entrance exam all those years ago – *Can someone else be a better judge of my interests than I am myself?* – and asked her how she would answer it today. Her response began emphatically, invoking the memory of her brother. "Yes," she wrote to me. "There is perhaps no better example of this than suicide. When people are in a suicidal crisis the brain functions differently. The rational thinking brain shuts down." But as her answer progressed, it became less emphatic and more qualified, until finally it gestured towards an acceptance of contingency.

"It's messy," she wrote, and it is – but mess is something she has spent a lifetime becoming much better at sitting with.

Afterword

You just got on with things, Peter once said. My father had said almost the exact same thing to me when I asked him, a few years ago, how he had once prepared for death when I was a boy and doctors had told him that the spread of his cancer was likely terminal.

At the time, my father had a wife and three young children, and his prospective death appeared to him as a logistical knot that he would untie for us in the time he had left. *You just got on with things* – but this rarely, if ever, meant talking about it.

Both my father and Peter can refer to extraordinary things in the most ordinary ways, and usually only after prompting. They are both very practical men, but they also share a modesty that seems so extreme as to resemble self-effacement. In fact, one might go further. A psychologist, reviewing a draft of this book, stopped at Peter's statement that "I'd never get buried – I don't want to become a chore to others to visit and remember". It expressed a fear of being burdensome, the psychologist said; a desire to minimise oneself. "In a way, he seems to be saying, 'I'm willing to be forgotten'," they told me, and this, too, reminded me of my father.

This wasn't the only similarity. When Peter spoke about his family history, and the various traumas buried within it, I was reminded of my own. On my father's side, it was also a family history of beaches and national service; prescribed social roles, unrecognised traumas, and serious wounds suffered wordlessly – a kind of scar tissue, I thought, that furled faintly through generations.

–

I have only one memory of my grandfather. It's modest and impressionistic, but sufficiently violent to have stayed with me. As a young boy – about four or five – I visited him at his beachside flat in which he lived alone, just across from the golf course he loved and on which he once scored a hole in one. There was just the three of us: my grandfather, my father and me.

The apartment was small, curiously furnished and bleached with sunlight. The meeting quickly dissolved into profane accusations, a loud and frightening exchange that ended with a slammed door and our hasty departure. That slammed door punctuated my time with my grandfather – I never saw him again before his death, in 1992, when I was eleven. I have no memory of his funeral, and my father has no memory of me attending, which almost certainly means I wasn't there.

Only much later did I realise that they were estranged, and that our visit had been an attempt by my father to force an introduction of at least one of his children to his father – who, it turned out, did not care for one. Apparently, my grandfather began tearing up his own wedding photos in some inexplicable spasm of rage, and then brazenly confessed his indifference about me. "I don't give a shit about you or your kids," were the last words I heard from him, my father said.

Forty years earlier, in a letter dated 17 September 1945, my grandfather wrote to his parents after his liberation from the Japanese camps where he'd been interned for three and a half years. "You've no idea how much I have missed Mel [my father] and Jean," he wrote, referring to his son and wife. "All the time I have tried to picture just what Mel looks like, but somehow I can't. He must be a lovely kid and I am breaking my neck to catch a glimpse of him. I hope he will know me from the photos Jean has of me. I don't know whether I have changed much, perhaps I have aged a bit."

I can remember returning to the apartment after his death and searching his drawers after being told that I could claim one small item. I chose a compass with a wrist band, given to my grandfather upon his enlistment, but, oblivious to its significance, I was entrusted with it for only a day.

The very few facts I knew about my grandfather, in lieu of a relationship with him, existed in my mind like deflated balloons from a long-ago party I was never invited to. I had to imagine the movement and noise – the *life* – that had once flowed around them.

One of those facts was that my grandfather's ashes were spread by his children across the eighth hole of the Seaview golf course, the site of his singular triumph. His children made their outlawed pilgrimage at night, and this defiance has always seemed charming and faintly heroic to me, principally because it was so uncharacteristic of my ultra-conforming father.

In January 1941, my grandfather was a travelling soap salesman for Lever Brothers. He was twenty-four years old and on weekends played footy for the West Perth reserves in the West Australian Football League. His wife would soon become pregnant with my father, but months before his birth my grandfather left for training in Darwin before being shipped to the front in Malaya. Before he was, he was allowed a trip back to Perth where he briefly met his newborn son – my father.

Some more facts: My grandfather enlisted on 18 January 1941. His Army ID was WX-15838, and he was a member of the 2/4 Machine Gun Battalion, A Company, 6 Platoon. The battalion comprised some 900 men, mostly West Australians, and by the time the Japanese surrendered, a little more than four years later, half of them would be dead.

My grandfather's battalion landed in Singapore in January 1942. In his first letter home from the front, he described to his parents the city's "magnificent buildings" built for "the moneyed people" and the hustle of the poor. He described cars and trains torn by shrapnel, and how the Japanese bombers would maintain high altitudes and then "drop their eggs altogether" while the boys "scramble down under cover in trenches and tell dirty yarns".

His battalion's journey to the Malaya front was longer than its engagement there. But the fighting they did was intense. Before Singapore fell to the Japanese in February, 137 men of the 2/4 Machine Gun Battalion were killed in action; the rest were marched off to prison camps. Now, my grandfather had another identifier: POW #1/12032.

A newspaper article from 31 August 1943: "First news of her soldier husband received by Mrs J.L. McKenzie-Murray in 19 months is an Army telegram informing her that he is a prisoner of war."

For the next three and a half years, my grandfather occupied multiple camps and hospitals. He was beaten, starved and forced, at the end of a gun or a whip, to carry and lay the sleepers of the Thai–Burma Railway. He suffered dysentery and malaria, and watched the decapitation of friends. Their heads were impaled on stakes – left as a warning or an obscene boast. Others died from disease, septic wounds or malnutrition.

After his liberation, he wrote to his parents again before embarking on the long journey home: "After a terrific day on the railway from five in the morning till eleven or twelve at night, in rain, mud and disease … you would arrive in camp to find your best mate had died while you were away at work."

Only much later, when I was an adult, did I realise the importance of music to my grandfather. In the camps, he kept a diary of sorts – a small book made from bartered paper, which he had bound with a vine and maintained at great personal risk. It contains descriptions of atrocities – one page is given to the severed heads – as well as the remembered lyrics of popular songs, their guitar chords and illustrations of their finger placements.

In another letter home in September 1945, my grandfather described singing in the camp, "not because I had any idea I could sing, but simply because it made others sing and they forgot some of the pain and sorrow. Even when I was sent to a hospital in Burma where only about one in five of us came out, I still sang my way through."

Twenty years later, my grandfather torched the rock music memorabilia obsessively acquired by his other son, my uncle, in the backyard of their home. In 1960s teen culture, my grandfather saw not pleasure or creativity, but indulgence and moral dissolution. The bonfire included a Kinks setlist, Roy Orbison's belt and Mick Jagger's harmonica – the last two items personally gifted to my uncle by their owners, and the first a souvenir from his time directing the band's stage lights on their second Australian tour. His vinyl collection and leather jackets were also added to the pyre.

"Dear Mum and Dad," my grandfather wrote from Singapore on 16 September 1945. It was his first letter home since his captivity began more than three years earlier. "It seems centuries since I have been able to sit down and write to you and now the opportunity has arrived I hardly know what to say."

But in two letters, written on consecutive days, he found things to say. Mostly expressing his wish to see his parents, his wife and the child he'd only fleetingly met before he shipped to Singapore. He wrote about his desire to enjoy the keg of beer his father had promised to celebrate his return. He described the letters to the dead that were still arriving from families yet to be notified of their deaths. And he wrote that "today, I got amongst a few [detained] Japs ... and believe me I subjected them to some of the humiliation they have taken so much delight in casting upon us during these three years of subjugation.

"The boys are arriving back to camp with all sorts of things including Japanese swords, revolvers, bayonets and heavens knows what not. Personally I am not bothered about souvenirs, the only one I am ambitious about bringing home is myself."

My grandfather hoped his repatriation would occur by plane, but it took two ships and a train, and weeks passed before he got home to his family and the keg of beer. But return he eventually did, and after the keg was emptied and the stories told, my grandfather took his wife and young son on a brief holiday in Perth's hills before going back to work. Lever Brothers had retained his job, but with a twist: it was now all regional work. And so, not long after his return, and without any form of counselling, he went to flog soap in the bush. He was home only every second weekend. "Those guys came back from war and just went back to their jobs after a couple of weeks' holiday and got on with it," my father says now. "There was nothing for them. There were a lot of suicides after that."

A resonance: some forty years later, my father was given a death sentence – advanced melanoma – and doctors told him to prepare his will. When I saw my skeletal father in a hospital bed, he looked like an intubated Pompeii victim. Remarkably, however, Dad survived. And when he returned home, he seemed as gently resigned to life as he had been to oblivion. There was no transformation, no *carpe diem*. He spent no more or less time with his children. He didn't take a lover, start a memoir or trek across Nepal. He filed his will away in the study and, much like his father, went back to selling insulation door-to-door. You just get on with things.

Five years after my grandfather's return from the camps, his wife was dead of a brain tumour. "Dad just sort of disappeared then," my father remembers. Dad and his younger brother were taken into the care of relatives for six months.

Two years later, my grandfather remarried. It was the same year one of his mates from the camps, recently released from Perth's repatriation hospital, stood in front of a train. A newspaper article, from 21 May 1952:

> After parking his car with its engine running a few yards away, John Alderton, single, French polisher, of East Street, Maylands, stood on the railway line at the Central Avenue crossing, Maylands, yesterday morning, and was struck by a north-bound train and killed.
>
> The driver of the locomotive, John McCaughey, of Sexton Road, Inglewood … said he could not stop the train in time and that as it approached the man put his hands across his eyes and stood facing the engine.

My grandfather never discussed such things, and my father never asked – not about the war, or the death of his mother, or his father's disappearance thereafter. There was no language for such things, and for generations the tongues of the men in my family were as dry as the bush in which my grandfather hawked soap after the war. *You just get on with things* was a personal code and respected ethic – and this form of stoicism could derange private suffering. Because if anguish and trauma had no language, they still found expression: in drink, in rages, in sullen retreats and unexplained vanishings. The trauma of war veterans was still largely regarded as a frailty of personality.

It was a bad deal. To have served the country, and then, having returned, to have to performatively disguise its costs. By interpreting trauma as personal failure, how many families were denuded of intimacy or of their capacity for tender curiosity? And for how many were these lessons internalised, normalised and transmitted through successive generations?

Well, I'm not sure you could count them all.

–

The generational transmission of trauma, and its influence upon their careers and self-conception, has long been accepted by Brett and Tara, who, with varying confidence, can plot some of the co-ordinates of that influence on their own life. Peter is more fatalistic and adrift from the meaning of his own past. "It's following us," he said to his young wife when Chernobyl's radioactive cloud drifted across Europe.

Like Brett and Tara, Peter saw the world as terribly unstable, and his strongest instinct was to impose order upon it. This need for control, of taming chaos, well preceded his PTSD – its onset only cruelly intensified it.

Of the three, Tara is conspicuous for having learnt to accept – and even find enthusiasm in – irresolution and uncertainty. She has melted her sword down, and when she came to eulogise her father, she could recognise the sorrow and disorder of his life alongside its love and humane ambitions – she could at once be sad and grateful, without the bruising oscillation between love and anger. Tara moved from domestic chaos to professional structure to learning to comfortably sit with the messiness of uncertainty and irresolution. In doing so, she may have escaped the existential jeopardy of depending upon something impossible – perfect control and certainty – for the maintenance of self-esteem. Of the three, Tara is perhaps the only one no longer intimidated by silence.

If Peter and Brett had inherited a blokey reticence that was reinforced by the culture of their work, then their participation in this book has, happily, thawed some of it. In September 2025, Peter texted me to say that he had shared his section with one of his sons – a young man who never quite knew the scale of his father's work, modestly concealed as it was, but who now "wept with pride" as he read about it.

Around the same time, Brett called me to share a modest breakthrough with his semi-estranged brother, Adam. Having read Adam's recollections of their time in the orphanage, Brett was naturally stung by the part in which Adam described his older brother as being far less protective than Brett would care to remember. It didn't quite accord with Brett's memories, but a conciliatory message was sent – one that led to a long-overdue phone call.

I was initially reluctant to include this detail, and not merely because it might appear self-congratulatory. My writing about these three lives in some way affected them. I was not only a sympathetic audience, but also a stirrer of things – and it was never guaranteed that such stirrings, however innocent, might not lead to further anguish. That the book encouraged these connections is wonderful, but only serves to remind me of the power of outside meddling and how badly it might've gone, too.

Then again, to neurotically twist myself once more, I'm reminded by a psychologist that people are often more resilient than we anticipate – and we shouldn't vainly expand our sense of care to a point that eclipses its object's agency and desires. "Curiosity about another's life doesn't usually go badly," the psychologist said.

And so, I hope, it is.

—

I've come to think of the work of the emergency worker as happening within a shadow world. Their world is braided with ours, but their work is such that the awful mess of accidents and violence are sufficiently cleaned that we only ever know them peripherally.

Let me tell you another story, an exceptionally strange one that was shared with me by a senior officer when I worked at Victoria Police. He could never forget, he told me, the time when he attended a house as a young officer, following a call about a drowning in a domestic pool.

As he approached the house with his partner, they were surprised to hear music. There was a party still happening – a middle-aged birthday. When they knocked on the front door, they were received by an embarrassed host who immediately began apologising for the noise. She invited them in.

The two officers exchanged a puzzled glance: *what on Earth was happening here?* They were there because her husband had been reported dead, but it was dawning on them now that no one had relayed this fact to her.

As they entered the house, they saw other revellers oblivious to the scene out the back. No one beside the pool had wanted to tell the dead man's wife, or anyone inside. And so, upon arrival, the officers found a bizarre partition that they would now need to collapse. They asked for the music to be turned off and went outside, where they confirmed the man dead. The scene was surreal and unsettling. It was the officers' duty to introduce those happily oblivious inside the house to the shadow world outside it. And it was their duty because those at the scene had outsourced the responsibility.

That moment is surely unrepeatable. But a recurring, extreme example of this shadow world – of work we outsource to obscure rooms and rarely consider – can be found with those who investigate child sex crimes. I had once thought that these duties might form a major part of this book, but I'm increasingly aware of the personal cost of writing such stories. Where once I was proudly unaffected, now there is usually some mental and visceral sickening. Undoubtedly, a major part of my vulnerability was becoming a father; upon reading about the abuse of children, my own daughter is instinctively invoked.

The same effect, magnified, can afflict first responders. I've heard many stories, while researching this book and beyond it, of first responders whose nervous collapse followed a personal association between a young victim and the responder's own child. We saw this in Peter's experience at Port Arthur. For those officers who examine child pornography for evidence, the risk is especially acute.

Many years ago, a police officer told me about this work. If a suspect is arrested and a cache of child pornography found, those images will usually show the abuse of different children by other offenders. A terrible door is then opened to much broader abuse, and these images must now be analysed for clues to the identity of both the victims and perpetrators. Thousands of profane images must be studied: what does the room's furniture reveal about their location in time or geography? Does this child's face, or clothing, correspond with other images we have? What detail can be lifted from the photo's metadata?

There was a rotation system for such work, and a psychologist was always present. But to carefully study such material – to examine images that would poison your faith in the very humanity that you've volunteered to protect – requires an awesome detachment. And to distance yourself from this obscenity is to risk detaching yourself from much else besides.

Most of the time we're protected from the shadow world. Tragedy or violence might visit us, but mostly we're shielded. The emergency worker isn't – the shadow world is their workplace.

–

When I spoke with Peter, I often thought of Ernest Hemingway and his time as a Red Cross ambulance driver during the First World War. I think of this still – not merely the facts of Hemingway's experience but also his intolerance of psychobiographers searching for meaning in it. "You do not like to be tailed, investigated, queried about, by any amateur detective no matter how scholarly or how straight," Hemingway wrote to a prospective biographer, the scholar Charles A. Fenton, in 1952, in what would be the first of several attempts to dissuade Fenton from his work.

Hemingway was only eighteen and had barely arrived in Italy when, in 1918, an explosion at a munitions factory just outside Milan obliged his attendance and transferral of dozens of body parts. "In the barbed wire fence enclosing the grounds and 300 yards from the factory were hung pieces of meat, chunks of heads, arms, legs, backs, hair and whole torsos," Hemingway's partner that day, Milford Baker, would later write in his diary. "We grabbed a stretcher and started to pick up the fragments. The first we saw was the body of a woman, legs gone, head gone, intestines strung out. Hemmie and I nearly passed out cold but gritted our teeth and laid the thing on the stretcher."

Only weeks later, Hemingway's legs were shredded in a mortar blast, and he recovered in a Milanese hospital – an episode later transformed into one of the Nick Adams short stories, 1927's "In Another Country". It opens: "In the fall the war was always there, but we did not go to it anymore."

In 1952, the scholar Philip Young published a revised version of his PhD thesis on Hemingway's work, which Hemingway initially and energetically sought to prevent. I first read the book in 2003, when I found a second-hand copy in an antique store in Seoul, not far from the city's major US military base. It remains the best thing I've ever read on Hemingway, a lively, well-written examination of his work and prosecution of a basic case: that much of his work, not least the string of early, exceptional short stories, were about fear and overcoming it, derived from his original "wounds" of 1918.

But Young went further. Hemingway was obsessed with danger, impulsively rushed towards it, and in doing so accumulated catastrophic mental and physical injuries – he had volunteered for too many crucibles and scorched his nervous system in the process. (He was also, oddly for a man who had courageously distinguished himself in various ways, an inveterate liar and exaggerator of stories regarding his physical heroism.)

As it was, Hemingway despised the intrusions and theories of scholars, none more so than those bearing Freudian analysis. In his foreword, Young tells us that his reluctant, increasingly indignant subject wrote to him: "To tell a writer he has a neurosis . . . is as bad as telling him he has cancer: you can put a writer permanently out of business this way."

In 1954, the year Hemingway won the Nobel Prize for Literature, he told *Time* magazine: "How would you like it if someone said that everything you've done in your life was done because of some trauma? I don't want to go down as the Legs Diamond of Letters." Jack "Legs" Diamond was a prohibition-era bootlegger who survived several assassination attempts. Hemingway did not want to be thought of merely as some plucky survivor, nor a sad captive to his so-called "traumas".

Hemingway's mental health only worsened, and Young's book found sharper light after his subject's suicide in 1961. In 1954, Hemingway experienced two consecutive plane crashes. In the first, in the Belgian Congo, his small aircraft clipped a telegraph wire and went down. His liver and kidney were ruptured, his lower spine crushed, his skull smashed open. His anus leaked, he saw double for a time, and he suffered temporary hearing loss. Almost implausibly, the rescue flight crashed too, and the aircraft ignited on impact. Hemingway was severely burnt.

Months later, having received the Nobel Prize – which he was not well enough to accept in person – Hemingway gave a sad, peculiar interview to CBS News, in which he relied upon cue cards for his answers. Watch it, and you'll see evidence of brain damage.

It's hard these days to accept Hemingway as a model for much. The man became terribly "truculent and childish", in the words of his final wife, and bitter and paranoid in the words of others, and for many years before his death he wrote in a funk of sickly self-parody.

In a Chicago blizzard in 2009, against the backdrop of similar thoughts, I walked between the Hemingway Museum in Oak Park and his childhood home a few blocks away. I'd taken the wrong train and thus endured a much longer walk to the museum than was necessary. Taking sympathy upon an Australian who'd surprisingly arrived in a snowstorm at this otherwise empty museum, the staff called ahead to Hemingway's childhood home to tell them not to close for the day because a young man was on his way.

Of 339 North Oak Park Avenue I recall very little, other than the sense that the man who let me in was the proud custodian of an American myth and unlikely to indulge my more complicated views of the man that I'd first encountered, aged twenty-one, in the short story "A Clean Well-Lighted Place".

That story was a revelation to me. In it, and in the others I read in the collection *The First 49 Stories*, I found subtle depictions of fear and trauma expressed with a musical plainness and made resonant by skilfully withheld information. The deep, melancholic suggestiveness of these stories reminded me then of how I received the occasional stories and whispered interpretations of my grandfather's time as a Japanese prisoner.

Later, I would come to find Hemingway excessively mannered and agree with the late critic Dwight Macdonald that the intensity of his austerity was always better suited to the short story. "It is curious how verbose Hemingway's laconic style can become," Macdonald wrote in 1962. And so it was, I thought.

I said none of this to the man who was so hospitably guiding me around Hemingway's shrine. Afterwards, we said goodbye and I returned to the blizzard outside, unsure what, if anything, I'd learnt by peering into these long-empty rooms.

Today, as I write this, I can see some things. My book's three exceptionally candid and bruised subjects each share something with Hemingway: an early, uneasy sense of inadequacy that was corrected by their assumption of public service and great risk. They ran into danger compulsively, to save others but also themselves. And it worked, until it didn't.

—

The clonidine means Peter rarely recalls his dreams now. But his wife can testify to his body's continued experience of them – he will still thrash about in the night. Before the clonidine, Peter dreamt of snakes and spiders, assembled in horrifying and impossible patterns. Now, the night trouble is largely Christine's.

Brett has two distinctive nightmares that he has experienced since childhood. One involves being chased by a grizzly bear. The other, he said, is more vivid. He's at his aunt and uncle's house in country Victoria, a place where he often spent his summer holidays from the orphanage. In waking life, the house was large to accommodate their eleven children and Brett told me that they always welcomed him despite the size of their flock. "Aunty Lenore and Uncle John's was my first real experience in a stable and loving family," he said. "I considered the children of this family to be more like brothers and sisters instead of cousins. Both Lenore and John were very good to me."

In the nightmare, a lion pursues him through the house.

I still have mine. The ones with the planes and the helicopters. My startle response in sleep has worsened recently, my partner tells me, and my night sweats have acquired an obscene quality: the smell of rancid meat. I suspect the recalibration of medication and the resumption of therapy may be wise.

Not unlike my three subjects, I too have been professionally drawn to trauma, and for reasons not entirely clear to me – not when it would make much more sense to quarantine myself, in so far as that's possible. To draw the blinds, milk my privileges and chase the frivolous. My pursuit of trauma has not been conducted in the same courageous manner as theirs, of course. Where they have rushed into fires, disarmed potential killers and performed rescues a kilometre beneath the earth, I have contented myself with contemplation. A poor comparison, then. But not, I think, a false or silly one. I've often thought of us as being on Fitzgerald's lonely boat, the one moving against the current, borne back ceaselessly into the past.

Acknowledgements

I'm indebted to the three major subjects of this book. *Sirens* doesn't exist without their trust, candour and respect for my independence – even if that independence might have caused them anxiety at times.

I'm also grateful to all the others who spoke to me, and mark here the memory of Simon Webb, who unfortunately did not live to see this work published.

The support of my partner, Stel, was, as usual, absolute. She was also a brilliantly perceptive reader, and in places both the shape and substance of this book were directly, and profitably, influenced by her. Merci, darling.

Heartfelt thanks to the team at Black Inc. – Sophy Williams and Denise O'Dea especially – whose talents unquestionably improved this book. I'm also grateful for their unerring patience regarding a manuscript that, for this reason and that, I seemed to forever be delaying the submission of. And thank you to Julia Carlomagno also, whose idea this book was some years ago.

Thanks also to my agent, Jane Novak, for years of warm, responsive and unfussy advocacy. There's no bullshit with Jane, and it's greatly appreciated.

Finally, I'd like to thank some friends. Richard Cooke and Andy Hazel for years of intellectual counsel and the lending of a sympathetic ear; and Ariane Beeston and Isabel Smith for their thoughtful and influential commentary on earlier drafts. This book contains the fingerprints of all four of you.